It's Like Heaven

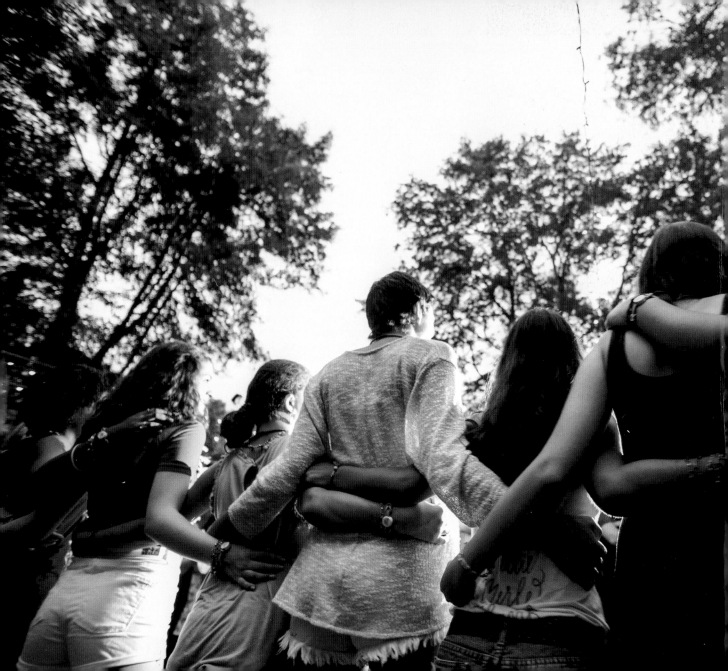

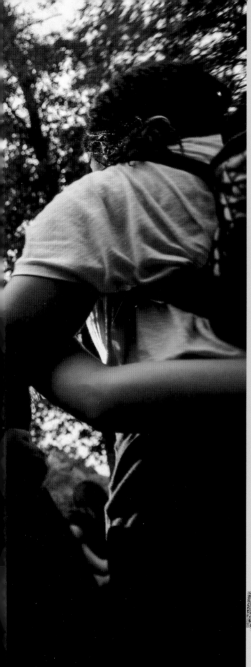

It's Like Heaven

STORIES FROM CAMP SUNSHINE

Edited by Dorothy H. Jordan

The University of Georgia Press   *Athens*

© 2020 by the University of Georgia Press
Athens, Georgia 30602
www.ugapress.org
All rights reserved
Designed by Erin Kirk New
Set in Minion Pro
Printed and bound by Pacom
The paper in this book meets the guidelines for
permanence and durability of the Committee on
Production Guidelines for Book Longevity of the
Council on Library Resources.

Most University of Georgia Press titles are
available from popular e-book vendors.

Printed in South Korea
24   23   22   21   20   C   5   4   3   2   1

Library of Congress Control Number: 2019957952
ISBN: 9780820357690 (hardback: alk. paper)
ISBN: 9780820357706 (ebook)

AUGUST 2020

This book is dedicated to every Camp Sunshine camper.

You have taught us more in a day than most can learn in

a lifetime about how to live and love, simply by sharing

your lives with us. I love you and thank you for the

privilege of being a part of your family.

—DOROTHY H. JORDAN

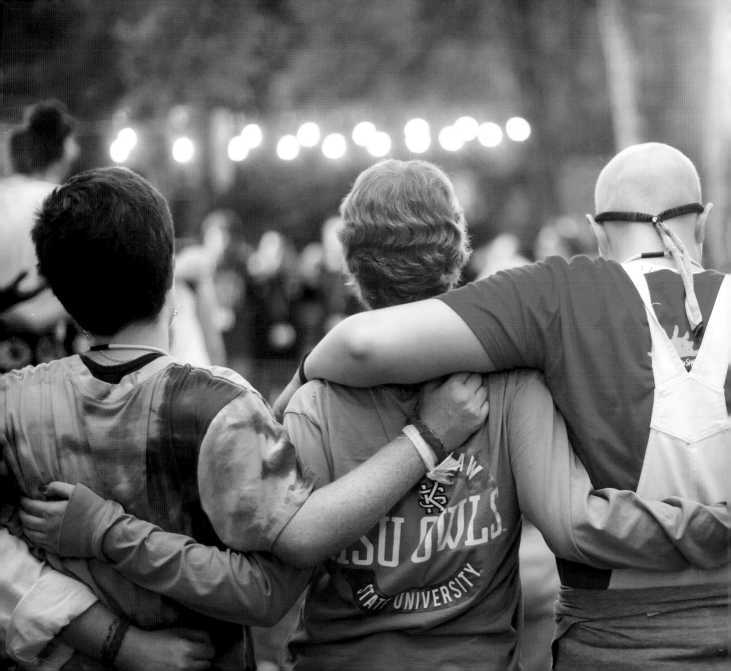

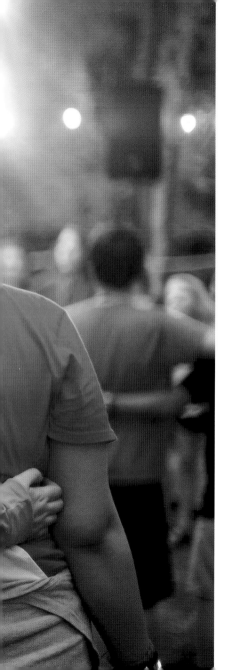

The connections we make in the course of a life—

maybe that's what heaven is.

—FRED ROGERS

Contents

Foreword

Karl Smart and Coach Kirby Smart

KARL

In the fall of 1989, I was fifteen and newly diagnosed with leukemia. I had just survived three awkward years of early adolescence. After a successful summer of competitive swimming, "two-a-days" of football practice in south Georgia, and my first Bainbridge High Football Training Camp at Troy State in South Alabama, I felt great! That fall I worked hard and played hard in the classroom and on the field, and I felt great. And then, I didn't.

It all happened so fast; I never saw it coming. I knew I was getting weaker but had minimal life experience to be truly alarmed. The day my labs were read, we left immediately for Tallahassee—the closest larger hospital. When we got off the elevator, I saw the name of the unit, oncology, turned to my mom, and asked, "Do I have cancer?" A day later this question was confirmed. I did.

On the way to a treatment center in Atlanta for a more extensive diagnostic workup, we stopped in Bainbridge to pack for what we figured would be a longer stay. I sat in the kitchen with my brother and sister. I knew they were scared just like my mom when we were in the hospital in Tallahassee. We were all scared. I tried joking with my brother, Kirby, about how I'd be back to full speed soon and would beat him in a sprint—even though he was always faster! I promised my mom I would beat cancer. But I was scared. Although afraid of cancer and afraid of dying, the care in their faces and the moments we shared in the kitchen that day made it clear I would fight with everything I had.

From the moment I entered the diagnostic and treatment phase at Egleston (now CHOA), I was hounded by nurses, doctors, and other patients about Camp Sunshine. I resisted for as long as I could. I'm generally an extrovert, but my experience of cancer felt too personal. Would going to camp make the pain my family and I were going through worse? Sometimes, yes. Would it be too awkward? At times, yes, but those sensitive moments changed me.

I was still a teenager, so meeting other teens with cancer would still be meeting other teens. Camp Sunshine was the place where I could flirt, dance, laugh, and cry. For a week, I could just be me. I could explore who I was like any other awkward pimple-faced teen. I didn't have to worry about how the gravity of cancer would impact others in conversation. Chemo jokes and late-night macho treatment stories about how it was making us ill became a rite of passage. Then came the friendships and losses that shaped my entire worldview.

When Dorothy first asked me to write this foreword in tandem with my brother, Kirby, I thought—what else is there to say about Camp Sunshine? Then I remembered my early days in the hospital and with my family. I remembered that this disease is *still* colliding with other kids' lives, like a comet! And I remembered that Camp Sunshine is still there, for them and for me and my family.

Last year, I moved with my family back to Georgia from California. I've been to camp three times since then. I have been a counselor in a cabin during teen retreat. I have helped tend to the Steve Davol Memory Garden and developed a stronger friendship with his sister, Lisa, and her family. And, I was able to visit on the day my brother, Kirby, brought the Dawgs to camp. I sat in the wings watching him tell a group of campers, counselors, and players how much Camp Sunshine has meant in our lives. I know my parents' burden was lightened knowing at Camp Sunshine I would have the chance to get more support and have fun, even in the midst of treatment.

It's tempting to forget how much cancer changed our lives and how painful it can be for survivors and families who've lost loved ones. Camp Sunshine keeps growing and changing. Holding on to the memories of the past, while developing innovative ways to serve more families and campers, through family retreats, the Camp Sunshine House, Remember the Sunshine events, and many other exciting new programs. Camp is alive and well, still helping kids and families make it through the dark times. There is so much more to say about Camp Sunshine! Forever let the sun shine on!

I was thirteen when my older brother, Karl, was diagnosed with acute lymphoblastic leukemia. I remember I didn't understand what that meant. I just wanted him to be OK. I do remember getting leukemia confused with Lou Gehrig's disease. I also remember sitting in our kitchen while Karl confidently told me he was going to beat cancer and how he was going to come back from it and beat me in a race. I'm happy to say that he was right on both counts.

Karl has an incredibly positive attitude, and I believe that if God had to pick who would have cancer and had to choose one person who was up to the challenge, it would have been Karl. My brother was hell-bent on winning this fight; there was just no way cancer was going to beat him. He was as brave as can be in the face of his diagnosis, but the battle was still tough on him and tough on our family.

My parents were juggling work, raising my sister, Kendall, and me, and doing everything they could to help Karl beat cancer. It was during this tough time that we saw the awesome power of community: the folks in Bainbridge who took care of my sister and me while my parents were taking Karl to get treatment in Atlanta; the doctors and nurses at Egleston Hospital who treated Karl and first told him about Camp Sunshine; and the counselors and campers at camp who embraced Karl when he got there and helped him to grow and heal.

Camp Sunshine is a refuge for kids with cancer. Being around other kids who had fought the same battle and won gave Karl hope; being challenged to try new experiences and meet new people gave him a piece of life he couldn't get at the hospital. Karl once told our mom that camp gave him a reason to live—a reason to keep going. Camp would eventually inspire Karl to keep spreading his hope to others as a counselor.

While Karl's camp experience is very special, I know it is not unique. I've had the opportunity to bring our football team to Camp Sunshine to visit with the kids for the past few years, and we've heard countless stories about people whose spirits were lifted and whose lives were changed by the commonality and love they found there. That's the special power Camp Sunshine has—a fellowship that drives people to volunteer their time to help give the next generation of young cancer patients and survivors the chance to heal and grow. And that same power drives my players to return to visit Camp Sunshine in greater numbers, year after year, looking to give back and be a part of this special community.

Bringing the players to camp doesn't just give the kids a memorable afternoon with their favorite Bulldog—it also gives our players an opportunity to learn how communities can empower others to overcome adversity. Seeing Karl battle cancer taught me a lot about resilience in the face of hardship, and I know that going to Camp Sunshine encourages our players to learn from these young campers about how to face life's challenges head-on. It can be a quiet drive from Camp Sunshine back to Athens as everyone counts their blessings.

In every corner of Georgia, I run into people who tell me about the joy Karl has brought into their lives through Camp Sunshine. That's not just a testament to Karl's big, loving personality; it's a testament to the camp's impact. Camp has given new life to Karl and so many others, and it has empowered them to pay that gift forward. Camp Sunshine has seen so many families like mine through their darkest hours by giving them a place to belong—a place to be a part of something bigger than themselves. I am eternally grateful for what the Camp Sunshine community has done for Karl and our family and what it continues to do for families across Georgia and the Southeast.

Acknowledgments

I am honored to have the opportunity to share a piece of Camp Sunshine. This book is a testament to the power of community, the remarkable Camp Sunshine community.

First, I'd like to thank all the book participants for sharing their stories. You are powerful, resilient, and inspiring.

Looking back, I realize that this has been a thirty-seven-year effort. To my late husband, Hamilton Jordan, I continue to feel your support, even in your absence from this place. I am grateful for all that we had together and have so many beautiful early Camp Sunshine memories with you.

My late parents, Dorothy and Russell Henry, who, I know, would be proud. They had a chance to hear about the early years of Camp Sunshine before their tragic, untimely death in 1988. I think of them daily and thank them for their unwavering love and support throughout my childhood and young adult life.

The Henry siblings, Tim, Sue, Nancy, and Rusty, thank you for loving me, your kid sister, always. Sue, I thank you for your eagle "English teacher" eye on this manuscript.

My children: Hamilton Jr., Kathleen, and Alex, you make me a better person every day. It has been my life's ultimate privilege to be your mother. Thank you for giving me the very best life role I could hope for and for always loving, inspiring, and supporting me. Alex, thank you for your excellent editorial assistance in the last drafts of the book manuscript.

Going back to the very beginning of Camp Sunshine, thank you Mo and Jane Thrash for your early and continued support, confidence in me, and support of Camp Sunshine. Mo, thank you for being our biggest

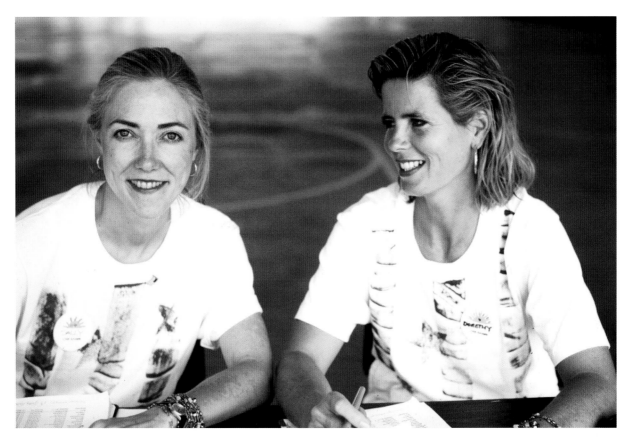

Sally (left) and Dorothy at summer camp, 1993

cheerleader, "preaching" about the power of Camp Sunshine to every single person you see, every day, without fail.

To all Camp Sunshine volunteers, the hundreds of you over the last thirty-seven years, what we experienced at our first camp in 1983 was the beginning of this magical thread that has stitched every one of us together. The strength of this connection is simply immeasurable, has changed lives, and will continue to do so. I thank you for your love and dedication to our campers and their families.

To the Camp Sunshine Board, thank you for your service to Camp Sunshine, your dedication to our mission, and your generosity. I thank the Atlanta philanthropic community for their continued and generous support of Camp Sunshine since 1982.

The impetus to write this book came in the fall of 2017. I was invited to join a few other Emory faculty at a small lunch gathering at the Carter Center with Pres. Jimmy Carter. The lunch conversation turned to writing books and Jim Grimsley, an accomplished playwright and novelist, and President Carter began discussing their latest publications. I was inspired by President Carter's writing accomplishments to get this book written! Thank you, Mr. President, for your love for me and my family and your support and encouragement.

I am honored beyond words. Jim Grimsley, thank you for your early advice and encouragement.

Both Camp Sunshine and this book would not be possible without Sally Hale, my dear friend and fellow nurse. Sally has been Camp Sunshine's brilliant leader as executive director for over thirty years. Sally, you know how much I lean on you in all areas of my life, and I am so very grateful for you, your friendship, advice, and constant support.

To Emory School of Nursing dean Linda McCauley and senior associate dean for academic advancement Sandi Dunbar, I thank you both for the opportunity to attend the School of Nursing writers' retreat in April 2018. This is where the book really began to gel and where I developed my plan to get this accomplished. Your support and confidence in me are so appreciated, and I am very grateful to be a part of your faculty.

Kylie Smith, you are a gem and I appreciate your mentorship, friendship, and excellent advice. I am so glad you came to us at Emory from "down under." I am also thankful for the friendship and support from our Emory book writing group. Your support and interest in this book have been a boost.

Camp Sunshine staff, thank you for your hard, dedicated work and all you do to keep our multiple programs running. I am grateful for you every day.

Tenise Newberg, you are the brain of all things Camp Sunshine. You are incredibly dedicated to Camp Sunshine, generous, and caring—your advice has been stellar.

Jeff Dunahoo, thank you for your assistance with photos; your superb talent and advice is very much appreciated.

Joan Kimble, thank you for your support, encouragement, brainstorming, and assistance with early planning and interviews.

Kenzie Mann, thank you for your excellent organizational and editorial assistance.

Thank you, Walter Biggins, for the opportunity to publish with you and UGA Press.

Finally, to my husband, Tom Grathwohl, I simply love you. We found each other because of our tragic losses and have forged a beautiful life together, and I am exceedingly grateful. Thank you for your constant, steadfast patience and support.

It's Like Heaven

Prologue

I'm a nurse. My very first job in high school was as a nurse's aide at a home for the elderly. I felt drawn to my patients, their stories. I *connected* with them and cared about them. This led to my degree in nursing and laid the groundwork for my full appreciation of the art of nursing. The most powerful tool we have as nurses and humans is ourselves, and sometimes the most healing action we can take is to just be there, to be *present* with the people we care for.

In 1982, as a pediatric oncology nurse, I saw a gap in care for children with cancer. Following a diagnosis of cancer and treatment in the hospital, children were often unable to find support in their home communities and felt isolated from their peers in between rounds of treatment and clinic appointments. I had a vision to fill this gap, a summer camp for children with cancer.

Forty-four children attended the first Camp Sunshine, a one-week summer camp in August 1983. In the early years, camp amenities were minimal, with a rustic cabin serving as the infirmary and sleeping quarters for me and my late husband, Hamilton. Today Camp Sunshine is a year-round resource for children with cancer and their families. In 2018, Camp Sunshine's thirty-fifth anniversary, more than 400 campers and 225 volunteers participated in summer camp. Camp Sunshine also has a permanent home since 2003, in Atlanta, where campers and families gather throughout the year for recreational, educational, and support programs. Camp Sunshine held 154 programs over 177 days during its thirty-fifth year with approximately 7,300 participants.

In 1983, thirteen-year-old Steve Davol was diagnosed with cancer. He was one of the original campers, participating in Camp Sunshine's first year. Steve had a magnetic personality and a passion for life, and though he died of cancer in 1997, his legacy lives larger than ever. At a young age, he understood the importance of the connections forged during camp and once described Camp Sunshine as "like heaven; everyone should go. But you have to be special—you have to have cancer." His story, as told by his sister, Lisa, exemplifies the connection that camp helps create; his words inspired the title of this book.

The story of Camp Sunshine is a powerful one of hope, love, and healing. It is the story of building a safe, caring, and inclusive community that embraces and inspires not only campers and their families but also the nurses, counselors, and other volunteers who care for them.

A contagious love

Steve Davol (April 5, 1969–January 7, 1997; hometown: Lawrenceville, Georgia), as told by Lisa Davol, and Tricia Benson

LISA

My brother, Steve, was diagnosed on a snow day in January 1983. We had no school, so it started off as a good day until he rammed his leg into a tree sledding down the neighbor's hill. Of course, we thought he had broken his leg because it swelled up so quickly. It's kind of amazing to think back now, though, that number one, we would have snow in Georgia and then that he would hit his leg on the tumor, which, had he not done, he may not have been diagnosed early enough for treatment.

Our parents took him to the hospital thinking he had broken his leg, and they ended up going straight to Egleston Children's Hospital. I just remember being at home with my neighbors. I knew it was bad because the neighbors were all concerned, and my mom was very upset once they found out what was going on. It felt like a whirlwind of *what do we do next* and *where do we go from here?* At that point, our family focused on how to get Steve the treatment he needed.

The family dynamic changed. It was a different focus. A lot of my childhood memories are of different points of his treatments or relapses or surgeries or whatever the case was. I was ten and Steve was thirteen when he was diagnosed. By the time camp rolled around that first year, a few months later, he had already turned fourteen.

That summer Steve was very hesitant to go to camp. He was reluctant to attend any kind of cancer camp. He was probably still dealing with the fact that he had cancer and maybe not wanting that label on him. But, when he came back from Camp Sunshine, that was when we started to see a positive change in him. Over

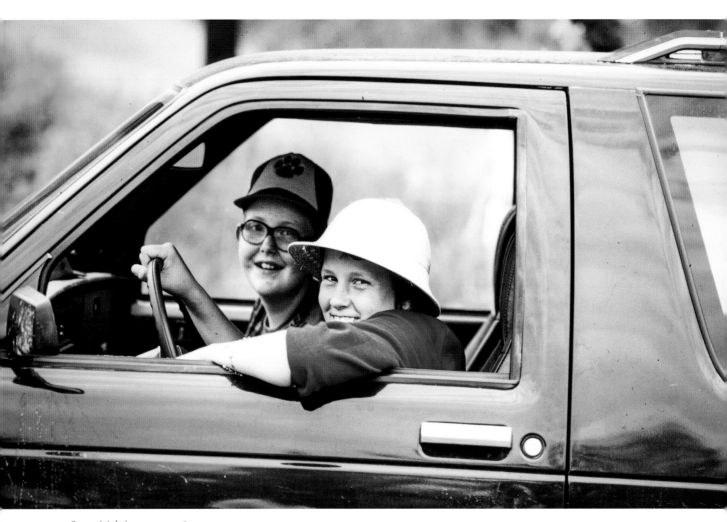

Steve (right), camper, 1983

the years, it continued. The more that he was involved with camp, the more hope he had. I think he just had a lot more joy and laughter, just understanding that he could live beyond cancer. It wasn't *yeah, I have cancer*, but instead, *I can still live beyond this. There's life beyond just having a cancer diagnosis.*

Camp completely transformed that whole diagnosis for him. Honestly, camp not only gave him hope but it gave him a lot of courage, and I think it gave him the will to keep fighting. Without Camp Sunshine, I'm not sure how his battle would have gone because I don't know that he would have had the same fight in him to live. It's powerful to think that one week at camp can do something like that for somebody. I remember watching the talent show with my family one year. It was so much of who Steve was. There he was "hamming it up" on stage, making everyone laugh, but truthfully, he was the one laughing the hardest, eyes twinkling mischievously. Camp Sunshine allowed Steve to be himself fully.

Steve had that magnetic persona about him. He had such a great, quick, dry wit and a lust for life. People were drawn to him. You couldn't help but be drawn to him. He just had that way about him. I read something in a book recently, a Maya Angelou quote, about how people will forget what you say. People will forget what you do for them and what you say about them, but people will never forget how you made them feel. Somehow, Steve drew people in, and he made them feel special. He made them feel loved.

Camp is the people. The activities are fantastic, and everything that Camp Sunshine does is amazing, but it's the people and how people make each other feel that is special. That's the impact being made. I think Steve epitomized that.

Steve's love didn't discriminate. Yes, he liked to stir the pot a lot and push the envelope. I've heard of more than one crazy camp prank he may have had a hand in, like the time camp woke up to a bike hanging from the high dive! I blame him if I ever am accused of "stirring the pot," too. That's his influence on me. He did it sometimes by picking on you but always in good fun. I remember Hamilton Jordan used to describe him as the Pied Piper. Kids were just drawn to him. You always knew that Steve loved you and he cared about you.

Camp Sunshine meant so much to him. When Steve was diagnosed, he automatically felt different from everybody else. There wasn't anybody his age in the community where we grew up that had cancer at that time. You feel kind of excluded because your life is so different and you're fighting this disease and you're the only kid in the school who is bald. But Camp Sunshine brought forty or so kids together with Steve. Cancer camp, I think, helped make cancer secondary because you were a kid first and your circle included everybody.

It didn't matter if you had a leg amputated or whatever the case was. Everybody was kind of the same at camp. I think about that connection, the impact that it's had on so many people. The ripple effect has just been amazing. I don't think you can even put a number on how many people have been connected because of camp. Camp has created a community, and it's truly like a family.

There's a kind of magic in watching these kids find the joy that they were missing or that fight to keep going or just not worrying for a while that they have cancer. They can make friends and be included and not be different. For some of these kids, it's a process to learn that and learn to be more inclusive with the other kids in their cabin. It's amazing how much they grow in a week at camp.

I am a counselor at Camp Sunshine now. This morning at breakfast, a senior camper announced, "This is my first year," and a big cheer erupted. Where else would someone get cheered on like that? You would think those "first-year" campers wouldn't feel so connected and such a part of camp because they haven't been there year after year. But no, everybody just embraces that like it's something to be celebrated. That's kind of how Steve looked at things. He said that having cancer may kill him one day, but it was never going to get the best of him. Yeah, cancer's a bad thing, but guess what? You've got Camp Sunshine and it's like heaven.

Steve felt that having cancer was a blessing in his life. How crazy is that to think that having a disease, a terminal one at that, is a blessing for you? I saw it at camp yesterday with one of the kids talking about how all these people get so worried and caught up about the little things. "Here I am battling cancer. You don't need to worry about the small stuff. You need to be positive." This is a child at cancer camp! I thought, *That's exactly how Steve would have said it.* "You don't need to be worried about these things. Look what I'm going through, and I'm still positive. I'm still living life." That energy and that love is awesome. It's like a contagious love that camp creates.

I think about how I decided to volunteer at camp after Steve died. Tricia Benson (former camp director and volunteer counselor) kept badgering me to go to camp. After Steve passed away, my family started going to the Remember the Sunshine weekends (bereavement weekends for families of campers who have died). Tricia asked me several times, "When are you coming to camp?"

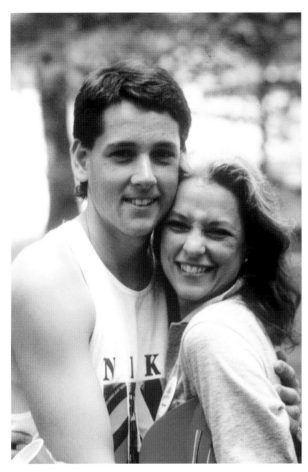

Steve at teen camp with counselor

I had worked at summer camps in college, and I was planning to work with kids as my career. It made sense for Tricia to ask, "Why don't you go to camp?" It took me awhile, though. I wasn't emotionally ready. Steve passed away in '97, and 2003 was my first year of volunteering. I gave myself about five years before I thought I could do it. The first summer there was rough. It was hard. I was just overwhelmed with the emotion of missing my brother.

For me personally, one of the beautiful things that I get to experience at camp is when twenty- and thirty-year volunteers come up to me and tell me stories about Steve. The stories were difficult to hear that first year at camp, but it's been a gift for me to be at camp and to hear them. Camp's like a family. You just feel embraced by everyone. There is so much support for me and that keeps drawing me back. You want to be part of the family.

Camp is a way for me to continue Steve's legacy. Even though he can't be here, I can still walk in his footsteps, although not exactly in the same way. I'm like any other volunteer here, though. Camp has given me more than I can ever give back. I think if you asked anybody who volunteers here, they'll say the same thing.

Today I'm the director for Oconee County Parks and Recreation. I want to do something in my life that

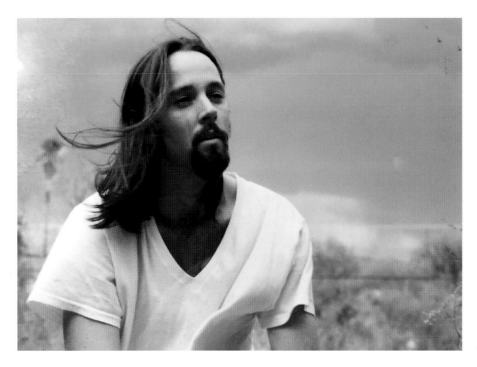

Steve (courtesy of Lisa Davol)

I love, that I enjoy, and that I feel has a purpose. I think it's something that Steve instilled in me, which was a big part of the impact he had on my life. I'm serving my community. My work has a purpose; it's something I have a passion for. I think it all goes back to camp and the impact it had on Steve. It impacted me, too, so that I want to live my life with a purpose and with a passion in whatever it is that I do.

Camp is a part of my life. I don't think I've missed a sibling camp since I first started volunteering. I try to participate in a family camp or a teen weekend and also try to schedule a day every fall and every spring to clean

Steve's garden, which Camp Sunshine completed a year after he passed away. It's important to me to keep the garden maintained for everybody else to enjoy, for it to be a nice, quiet place of reflection for anybody who goes to camp.

If Steve were alive today and meeting a newly diagnosed child, I think he would say, "You have to go to camp. You can't miss camp. You go once, and you'll always be back because you're going to have the time of your life."

It is amazing for a child that's just been diagnosed with cancer to know, *I can do something that's going to make me have the time of my life when I've got all this other crap going on.* The joy that camp can bring that child in just a week will carry them throughout the entire year. They'll hold onto that joy for the whole year, no matter what they're having to go through, what treatments they're having. Steve dealt with that because he relapsed over and over and over again. A number of Camp Sunshine volunteers are childhood cancer survivors and are such great role models for these kids.

Steve helped me be to be a wiser counselor—I witnessed his transformation because of camp. He was an above-the-knee amputee who had a third of his lung removed, yet he lived without limits. He kicked my butt on the tennis court. He snow skied. At camp, he climbed the climbing wall and high ropes course. It didn't matter what the activity was. In my eyes, it seemed he could do anything. He had been bald so many times that it didn't look different to me.

Because of Steve's attitude, I felt like there was nothing these children couldn't do. It was like, *So what that you have cancer? I don't care that you have cancer. A lot of people have had cancer. So what if you're missing a leg or an arm? Don't let that hold you back.* I know I got that attitude by living with someone who didn't have any boundaries. There was nothing holding him back.

The volunteers and former campers that go back year after year and bring that passion, keep it alive—that's magic. The kids going to camp don't have a choice! They're going to have a good time. We tell them, "We are going to change your life and impact you for the rest of your life. That's just the way it is." Campers come in, and we just know that this is what's going to happen. "We're going to do everything you can do at camp this week and then you're going to go home. But you're going to have an incredible year because you're always going to remember back to how camp affected you, and how you're not different. You can go out and make friends and do all those other things that kids

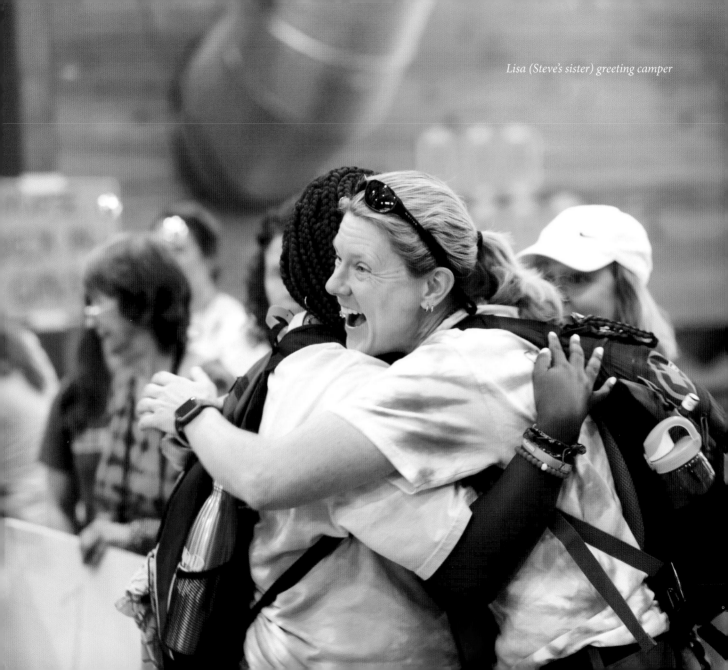

Lisa (Steve's sister) greeting camper

do. Cancer's just one of the many things that you have to deal with."

The people are what make Camp Sunshine special, who make meaningful experiences for these kids. Camp nurtures those relationships and keeps people engaged. That's the connection. It's the community that camp has built.

TRICIA

When I was in nursing school at Vanderbilt, I worked during the summer between my junior and senior year as a student nurse intern. During that summer I took care of a teenager with a brain tumor. I learned more from caring for her and her family over that summer than I did in all my classes. From that experience, I knew I wanted to work in pediatric oncology.

I moved to Atlanta in 1982 and began working on the pediatric hematology/oncology unit at Egleston Children's Hospital, now Children's Healthcare of Atlanta. I remember Dorothy Jordan coming to a staff meeting and sharing with us that she was starting a camp for children with cancer with the first session to be held in the summer of 1983. Dorothy was looking for volunteers, and I jumped at the opportunity. Several other nurses volunteered for that first camp—a tradition that continues today of extending pediatric oncology care beyond the bedside and the hospital setting to bunks in the camp setting.

Camp Sunshine that first year was magical—as it has been every year since 1983. The camp activities are so secondary to the love, hope, and support shared with campers and volunteer staff alike. I loved it so much, I became one of the camp directors for a few years—still one of my favorite jobs of all time!

Those first years of camp we leased space at other existing summer camps. High Harbor, Camp Coleman, and Camp Barney Medintz were much more rustic than Camp Twin Lakes, which we have used for the last twenty-five years. Camp Twin Lakes has allowed Camp Sunshine to serve not only more children but children who are weaker and need more support because of their disease and/or treatment. Building the Camp Sunshine House in 2003 provided a permanent home and the hub for all the work around the state.

In so many ways, Camp Sunshine remains the same as it was in 1983. The core—volunteers, dedicated medical team, strong professional staff, trusting parents, and, most of all, campers full of love, determination, grit, hope, laughter, friendships—does not change.

Camp has been part of my life for thirty-six years. I am not sure I ever go a full day without thinking of someone or something that reminds me of camp. My closest friends are camp people. The campers and families taught me how to live life to the fullest—and to love more deeply in the time we have together. I hug my children tighter because of the campers and families I have known.

Lisa Davol has been a volunteer for a long time now, but I met Lisa many years ago as the younger sister of Steve Davol. I was one of Steve's nurses. Lisa attended Camp Sunshine's sibling camp and later Remember the Sunshine, Camp Sunshine's program for bereaved families.

In my role as executive director with Camp Sunshine, I did a lot of volunteer training. I often shared a line for volunteers to remember: "*It's not your journey.*" I meant that a volunteer's time at camp should always be about the campers' experiences. Camp is fun for everybody. Camp counselors can get caught up in the moment of an activity—winning a softball game, showing off a new dance move, or catching the biggest fish. The priority of a volunteer counselor at camp must always be about the camper's journey versus their own.

We always must remember that parents trust Camp Sunshine to care for their children—and what is

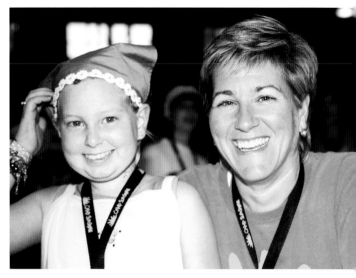

Tricia with camper

uniquely different is that these children may have limited days, weeks, months, or years to live. For parents to share a week is indeed a gift beyond measure. The emotional, physical, and spiritual safety of the camper is imperative in part because of the reality of childhood cancer. I am reminded of all the weeks Steve spent at Camp Sunshine—away from his parents and family. What a privilege. I am grateful to his family for sharing him with us.

The bond of campers to each other at camp and, by extension, to the children's families are far more important than the activities of camp. Because of that connection, I knew Lisa would be a great Camp Sunshine counselor. Because of that sense of community, I have witnessed and shared a deeper understanding of hope, courage, and love.

It is hard when we lose a camper, and over thirty-six years, there have been many losses. We grieve alongside the family. I wish I could tell so many parents, "I remember you and your child, and I thank you for sharing your child with us."

Steve embodied all that is Camp Sunshine. Now, Lisa volunteers in Steve's honor and memory, her presence adding another wonderful part of the rich Camp Sunshine fabric. Lisa, too, embodies all that is Camp Sunshine. Lisa loves camp as much as Steve loved camp.

Camp Sunshine is hard to put into words . . . *unconditional love . . . a sacred space.* . . . My best effort is just to quote Steve, *"It's like heaven . . ."*

2 I'll always be here for you

Montana Brown (born August 21, 1993; hometown: Columbus, Georgia) and Harleigh Sohler

MONTANA

It's often best to start at the beginning. So I'll start at the beginning of my childhood cancer journey. I was two years old at my first diagnosis. I don't remember much from that first battle with cancer. The nurses at Children's Healthcare of Atlanta told my parents about Camp Sunshine. Since I was only two years old at the time, I was too young to attend summer camp. So instead, my family and I attended a weekend family camp. My parents enjoyed that first Camp Sunshine experience, and when I was old enough to go to summer camp, I went.

I attended my first summer camp when I was seven years old, which would have been in 2000. According to my mom, I was really scared at first, but at the end of the week, when she came to pick me up, I didn't want to leave. That is a typical camp reaction, if you ask me.

At the time of my second diagnosis, I was fifteen years old and was at the end of my ninth-grade year in high school. It was only a couple of months before I was supposed to go to camp. I had just moved to a new town and tried out for the school cheerleading team (and made it!). I was also on a competitive cheerleading team.

First, I started noticing some fatigue and felt an overall sense of "something just isn't right." Since I was first diagnosed when I was younger, my parents took me to see one of my doctors from that time. I was diagnosed with rhabdomyosarcoma again. It's a soft tissue tumor—my tumor was in my abdomen. Unlike with my first cancer, I remember the second time. We were all extremely shocked. The doctors told us that it was very

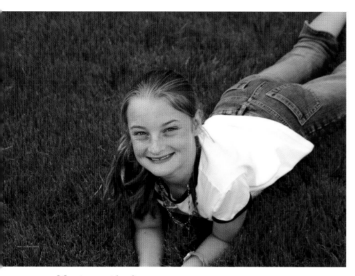

Montana at junior camp

rare for the exact same cancer to come back in the same spot almost thirteen years later. The first treatment course was a tumor resection and chemotherapy for one year. The second time I went through a tumor resection, chemotherapy for one year, and radiation for six weeks.

I was so nervous to go back to camp because no one knew that I had been rediagnosed. I had been getting chemo, I was weak, I was losing my hair, and I wasn't the same Montana that everyone had come to know over the previous years. Walking into camp on that first day, I was worried that people would treat me differently because of my new cancer diagnosis. As I entered the cabin full of girls I had grown up with, I was reminded of how camp is a not a place where you are treated differently simply because you have cancer. They each embraced me with hugs like they had done every year before. We talked, we laughed, and we had the same amount of fun as we had in the past. It was honestly such an amazing moment during my camp experience. Having that support during my second cancer diagnosis is a feeling I will never be able to explain. It truly meant the world to have the campers and staff by my side.

The Camp Sunshine community has meant the world to me for many reasons. Not only has camp given me lifelong friends, it's given me a place to call home. I know that no matter where I am at in life, I will always have Camp Sunshine to stand with me and be there for me. It's a safe haven, a place to run to when I am feeling sad, and a place to rejoice when I am happy. It's an endless support system that will stick with me for the rest of my life.

Camp Sunshine gave me my best friend, Harleigh Sohler. Harleigh and I met in 2012 during her last year at camp and my first year on staff at Camp Twin Lakes, where I worked during college for two years.

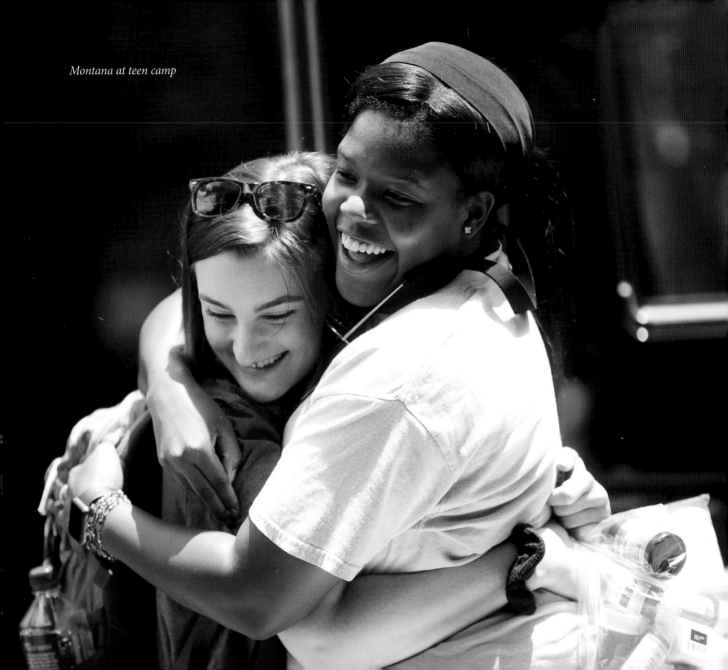

Montana at teen camp

A counselor introduced us because she thought we had similar personalities and would get along great. She was right. Harleigh and I hit it off immediately. I learned during that week that Harleigh was going to go to school at Georgia Regents University, the same college I was attending. I was so excited to have a fellow "Camp Sunshiner" in Augusta with me. After the week was over, our relationship continued to grow. She came to college in the fall and joined my sorority, and we ended up being big/little sisters. Having Harleigh in my life has been a blessing. She has been there with me through nursing-school tears and graduations; she was there for me when I got my first "big kid" job; she was there when I got my dream job at Children's Healthcare of Atlanta; and she's still here now. Harleigh has been a constant in my life since the day I met her. She is someone I can always count on, no matter what. Without cancer and Camp Sunshine, I wouldn't have her. I'm so grateful to the counselor who introduced us. She knew that we needed each other.

I was a camper at Camp Sunshine for eleven years and have stayed connected to its programs since graduating in 2011. I worked at Camp Twin Lakes and now volunteer at Camp Sunshine teen week and other camp events during the year. It feels natural to stay part of the camp family.

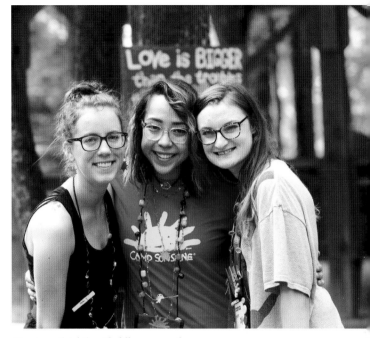

Montana (right) with fellow counselors

I tell new campers, "Don't be afraid to be yourself." I know that sounds like silly and stereotypical advice, but let me explain. When you first arrive at camp, it's easy to want to wear a "cool hat." You want everyone to think you are cool, so you don't participate in the goofy things that make camp, camp. We do silly things like beat on the tables, dance in the dining hall, and even make people shake their booty in front of the entire camp! If you keep your "cool hat" on and don't participate in these things, you won't get the full experience that camp has to offer. Camp is all about stepping outside your comfort zone. So, my advice? Do not be afraid to do just that.

I am currently a nurse on the Aflac Cancer and Blood Disorders Unit at Children's Healthcare of Atlanta—Scottish Rite. It's so amazing to be able to work in the same hospital that treated me as a child and teenager. As of right now, my plan is to stay there as a bedside nurse. Maybe one day I'll advance to be a nurse practitioner, but for now, I'm just happy for the amazing opportunity to fulfill my lifelong passion of taking care of children with cancer.

HARLEIGH

I had my first chemotherapy treatment in early June and my second chemo at camp. That's how fast it all happened.

I was diagnosed with an optic pathway glioma, which is a brain tumor, at the end of my freshman year of high school. I was fifteen and had made the football cheerleading team, and everything was going great. I was seeing an ophthalmologist because of a problem with my eyes; my great-grandmother had glaucoma, and my parents were worried that I would develop early glaucoma due to what my optometrist told us. After the optometrist shared that news, we were told to see an ophthalmologist so that my eye development could be tracked over the years. During one of my appointments, the ophthalmologist checked my peripheral vision, and the test came back completely black, meaning I missed everything. It was showing that I had no peripheral vision. The ophthalmologist was puzzled as he said, "I saw you six months ago, and your peripheral vision was fine."

Obviously, we knew something was really wrong. I had recently gotten my driver's license, and sometimes I would miss things when I was driving. My mom thought I was just being a bratty teenage driver who wasn't paying full attention, but it wasn't that at all. The ophthalmologist ordered an MRI, and two days later, my mom received a phone call saying that it showed a tumor on the right side of my optic nerves, just behind the chiasm. That's why I was losing my peripheral vision.

First, we met with a neurosurgeon who told us that I had an inoperable tumor and that the cons of trying

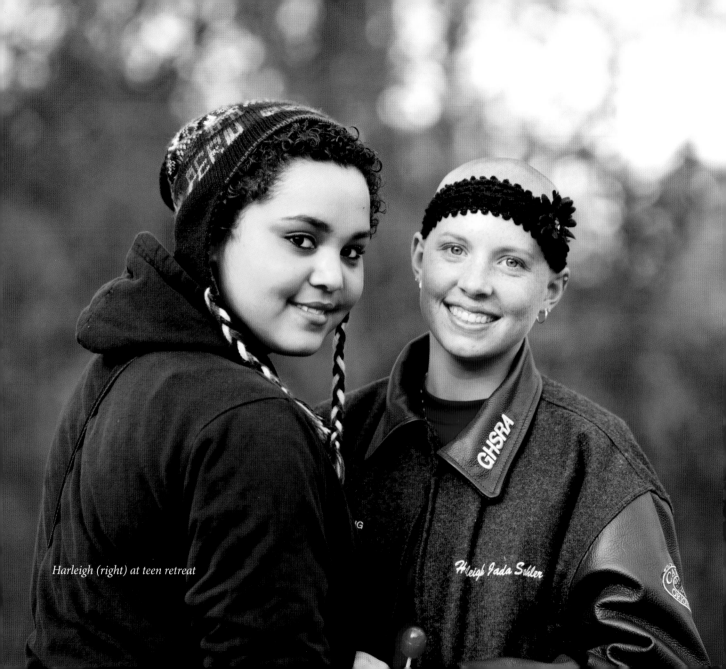

Harleigh (right) at teen retreat

to surgically remove it far outweighed the pros. That's when we were referred to an oncologist, Dr. Claire Mazewski, at the Aflac Cancer Center at Children's Healthcare of Atlanta. Dr. Claire is a genius and a godsend, and I love her. I had my first chemotherapy treatment in June, and because of my blood counts and other unforeseen circumstances, I ended up having sixteen months of chemotherapy.

I had my ups and downs during treatment. I had every known side effect and then some! At first, I really pushed myself. I would have treatments on Monday and then go to school Tuesday through Friday, but I was just wearing myself out. Then I started doing treatments on Monday, resting on Tuesday and Wednesday, and going to school on Thursday and Friday. I did that for a year and a half, but I kept up with my classes. There was one teacher who graciously stayed with me after school until 6:30 or 7:00 at night to make sure that I could keep up with my work; she helped me as much as she could. I even continued cheering, although toward the end of the season, I had to wrap myself up in blankets and sit out on the sidelines before the end of the games.

The timing of my diagnosis and initial treatment was insane. I met Dr. Claire at the end of May, and nearly right away, she told me, "There is this camp you have to go to, Camp Sunshine. It's for kids with cancer, and I think you should go." My immediate reaction was, *I definitely won't be going to that camp. I am not going to a camp to sit around all day and cry with other people. We get it: we've got cancer, our lives suck. What more is there to know?* My mom asked every question you could think of, but she was emphatic: "Oh, you're going!" I was not excited, to say the least.

My mom made me ride the bus to camp so that I could have the whole experience. When I arrived at Camp Twin Lakes, I was honestly shocked . . . but in a good way. There were so many people, and everybody was running up to people they knew and hugging them. I wasn't sure what I had gotten into, but I figured, *I'm here for a week, so I might as well make the most of it.*

I started walking to the cabin with the other girls, staying a little bit behind them, when all of a sudden, I started crying. I thought, *Everybody knows each other, and I'm going to stick out like a sore thumb.* I felt alone, and I missed my mom. One of the girls, Claire Hayes, stopped to wait for me. She said, "Listen, don't worry about it; we've all been there." I told her I was sorry, that I couldn't believe I was crying. She said, "Let it all out. We've all been there. We all get it, and that's why we are here."

Within the first twenty-four hours, I knew I was going to be OK. I was new to camp and new to the cabin, but everyone welcomed me. I told my cabinmates, "I know that I'm the new kid on the block, but please help me understand what's happening here. Please tell me everything I need to know." The eight girls and three women in my cabin were so supportive and so helpful to me. I remember we started off by playing an icebreaker game, and I thought it might be awkward; turns out, I was wrong. Everybody shared what they wanted to share—*this is who I am; this is how old I am; this is my diagnosis*. One thing I learned from that week at camp is that cancer is cancer. I might have a brain tumor and you might have leukemia, and while everybody has their own battle to fight, there is so much we can understand and share and learn from one another.

I can tell you that meeting Montana was one of those life moments when you just know, *this person is going to be my lifelong friend*. I think Montana felt the same way. She is a little older than me, so my first summer at camp was her last summer at camp. I didn't meet her when she was a camper. One day during my last summer as a camper, one of the counselors asked me where I was going to college. When I responded, "Georgia Regents University," she jumped up and said, "Don't

move. There's somebody you've got to meet." She ran out and came back with a brown-haired girl wearing a Camp Twin Lakes lanyard around her neck—it was Montana. It turned out she had been a Camp Sunshine camper, and she was currently going to Georgia Regents University. Montana had graduated from teen camp and was working on the Camp Twin Lakes staff for the summer. She was a sister of Alpha Delta Pi, and I had already known that I wanted to join ADPi.

We hung out together the rest of the week at camp. Camp is what made me so comfortable talking to Montana in the first place, and because of the relationship we formed at camp, I knew someone had my back before I even got to Georgia Regents University. When I started school, I went through the recruitment process, joined ADPi, and later became her "little" (sorority sister), so she was officially my "big."

The summer after my first year at college, I got the chance to work with Montana at Camp Twin Lakes. I got to spend twelve weeks with my very best friend. Of course, sometimes we wanted to kill each other, but it was great! I am a very emotional person, so Montana gave me a heads-up about working at camp. She warned me there would be times when I would cry, times when I would laugh, and everything in between. It is life changing to work as a counselor at a camp with kids with disabilities or serious illnesses. For me, being on the other side of the camp experience was incredible. I hadn't been out of camp very long myself at that point. I still knew campers there during Camp Sunshine week. It was a bit of a struggle for me to separate the two: camp and my job.

Today, even though I'm getting ready to graduate with my degree in social work and Montana is working night shifts as a nurse, we talk on the phone almost every morning. Montana just got engaged to a former Camp Sunshine camper!

Part of the whole childhood cancer scenario is that you learn quickly that you can't take life for granted; you can't miss a moment. Cancer taught me that if you have a gut feeling about doing something, then you'd better do it. If it's not in your comfort zone, that's all the more reason to do it. It took the biggest leap of faith for me to go to camp, but no exaggeration, the people I met saved my life. I would not be where I am today or who I am without camp. There are still so many people I stay connected to from Camp Sunshine, and even if we haven't talked or seen each other for a while, we never skip a beat. When I think about the people I've lost, I am so glad to have known them and to have reached out to them and to have had them in my life. I never thought these connections I have with people from camp could be so strong and so real. Almost everyone has people in life who say, *I'll always be here for you*. But at Camp Sunshine, when someone says that, that person really means it.

3

A feeling that's hard to beat

Kevin "Vinnie" Skelly (August 20, 1979–August 30, 2019; hometown: Roswell, Georgia), John and Carlene Parker, and Jane Clark

VINNIE

I was five when I was diagnosed with acute lymphoblastic leukemia in 1984. My parents had enrolled me in a soccer league, which was fine, but they couldn't understand why I wasn't interested in it, why I wasn't running around the field like the other boys, why my body was hurting, and why I was sore all the time. They thought maybe I had injured myself, but I hadn't, and we could find no explanation. They took me to a doc-in-the-box to have it checked out. The doctors did preliminary blood work and sent it off to be evaluated. I remember their reassurances telling my parents there was probably nothing to worry about. Within three weeks, the results were back, things didn't look good, and I was seeing an oncology team at Scottish Rite Children's Hospital in Atlanta.

Basically, my blood test showed that my leukocytes were blasting off the charts. I remember the doctors telling my parents, "A normal blood cell count is this, and your son's is eight times that number." So in November 1984, on my dad's birthday, my dad learned his second-youngest child had leukemia. *Happy birthday, Dad*, right?

I can remember being in the hospital throughout the Thanksgiving and Christmas holidays. I was in the hospital for twelve weeks. I think I had a break at New Year's. I remember Santa Claus visiting the floor; I have an old Polaroid photograph of Santa Claus and me that's lost all its color by now. I think I was being a grouch, not so much grouchy about missing Christmas at home but more about the food in the hospital!

My treatment continued into 1985. Because of treatment and hospitalizations, I ended up joining kinder-

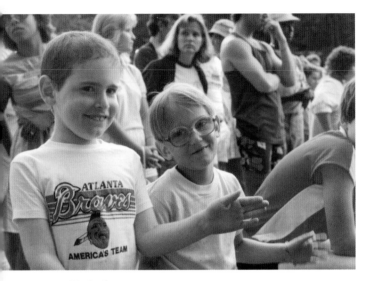

Kevin, first year at camp

The following year, in 1986, I was old enough to attend a camp for kids with cancer called Camp Sunshine. Sally Hale, a nurse at the pediatric oncology clinic and part of the medical team that treated me, first told my family and me about Camp Sunshine. I attended my first summer camp in 1986. I was hooked!

For thirty years, I never missed summer camp. I participated as a camper until graduating from high school and then became a counselor in training and finally a volunteer counselor. In 2016, I faced yet another acute lymphoblastic leukemia diagnosis and had to miss summer camp for the first time as I fought cancer all over again, this time as an adult.

My wife, Kelly, and I knew something was wrong. I started coming home from work feeling terribly fatigued and with unexplainable bruises. Doctors determined that I had leukemia again. My diagnosis was related to having a specific abnormality (the Philadelphia chromosome) that they weren't testing for in 1985 when I was diagnosed. I began a treatment protocol of radiation and chemotherapy. But unlike in the 1980s, due to advancements in medical technology and cancer treatment, I was advised that my best chance to beat leukemia this time and achieve remission was a bone marrow transplant.

garten a little late. I was still on active treatment even as I was going into first grade. It wasn't a great time for me. I had a central line (also known as a port—a surgically placed catheter on the chest, allowing for chemo administration and blood draws, decreasing the number of needle sticks); I wasn't allowed to do certain activities. And I was still bald and had a hooded sweatshirt on all the time. I still kept falling asleep in Miss Langford's class and not understanding why!

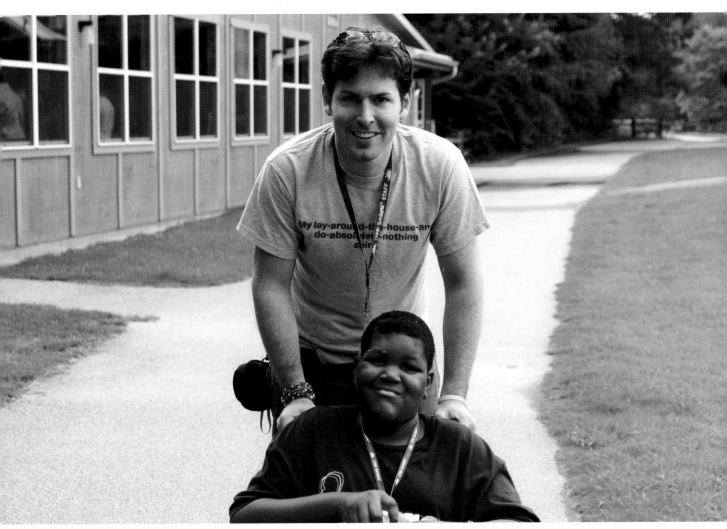

Kevin as counselor

By the grace of God and really great genes, I learned that my older sister, Sharon, was a donor match. A sister-to-brother match is rare in bone marrow transplants. But they looked at ten markers to determine a match, and each of the markers they looked at—*every single one*—was a perfect match with my sister. I remember my wife, Kelly, calling a family meeting to let everyone know. She said, "We have some really great news. Sharon is a perfect match."

My sister, Sharon, is about ten years older than I, so when I was diagnosed as a kid, she had a front-row seat for all that my diagnosis and treatment entailed. So now here we were in 2016, and she was front and center again as my perfect donor match! My bone marrow transplant was done at Northside Hospital, Atlanta, and I achieved remission in the fall of 2017.

Camp Sunshine's incredible network of competent and compassionate people was a tremendous blessing not just to me as a kid with cancer and a camp volunteer but now, again, as I was facing this second cancer. Because of my previous diagnosis and being surrounded by survivors at Camp Sunshine, getting the adult diagnosis was not as scary as it might have been. Certainly, it was a sock in the gut, and yes, it did scare me for a day or so. But having faced this disease before, I knew a lot more about what to expect—and I knew what resources were available to me.

Included in that circle of friends are John and Carlene Parker, volunteer counselors from my days at camp. They are great people. John was my first cabin counselor. He is the one who got me to come out of my shell at camp. He also was my guide and mentor when I became a new volunteer counselor. You know those people you meet in your life who can be over-the-top singing your praises and, at least in your own opinion, end up overselling you? John was great at that—he was like my biggest fan, a cheerleader. Always.

So many people impacted me on my journey, but Jane Clark is beyond wonderful! When I got my diagnosis in 2016, she was one of the first people I called. I said, "Hey, Miss Jane. It's Vinnie from Camp Sunshine. You'll never guess what I did. I just got myself leukemia again."

From that point on, Jane was an incredible resource for me. I looked to her for input and expertise on which cancer center I should turn to for treatment. Basically, she said, "Tell them I sent you. I've worked with all the nurses on the floor and all the oncology doctors. I know them. They are excellent." Talk about putting your mind at ease! For someone in my position, it was incredible to have a network of individuals to guide and support me. The friends and relationships I developed through Camp Sunshine equipped me for adult cancer. Who else has been blessed like that?

When I went to camp for the first time, I was a shy and afraid boy. I didn't know anyone. I was a kid with cancer; I didn't know any of these other kids. Then the next thing I know, here comes Jane Clark, who popped out the acoustic guitar and taught everybody the peanut butter and jelly song, and suddenly, we're all on a level playing field. It was beautiful.

It's phenomenal to think that camp has produced a whole group of people who work so beautifully together to make things less scary and more positive for kids battling cancer. Jane Clark has touched this disease so profoundly. Not only is this her life's work, but she also gives two weeks of her time every year to Camp Sunshine. She is a volunteer; she does not get paid to do this. She is undercelebrated as are all pediatric oncology nurses.

My wife, Kelly, and I met at camp and were married in 2006. We're celebrating twelve years of marriage and we have three little ones at home. Our son Liam was born in 2010, followed by our second son, Everett, in April 2012. Kelly understandably had to step away from camp after our first child was born, but we still felt it was very important for one of us to stay connected.

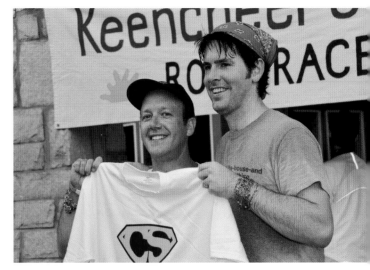

Kevin (right) with fellow counselor

One of my sweetest family memories of Camp Sunshine is summer camp of 2012, not long after baby Everett's birth. Kelly and I took the boys with us, and I remember Sally Hale greeting us when we arrived—it was special to have my family go to camp. Kelly, with baby Everett in her arms, and Liam came to my cabin. They all helped me make my bed and got to see where Daddy would host a group of boys for a week—be their camp counselor. It was just a special time. A few weeks after that, Everett died unexpectedly. It was an unspeakable loss. But I am so thankful to have that memory—that Everett was there with me at Camp Sunshine.

Following Everett's sudden death at just three months old, Sally Hale, the executive director of Camp Sunshine, and Tenise Newberg, the program director, showed up at my mom and dad's house in Marietta where everyone was gathering, bringing food and beverages. Without waiting to be asked or asking what they could do to help, they just moved right in and took care of things. I remember Sally talking to me and reminding me that her grandfather's name was Everett, and she shared the memory of seeing the boys tucking me in at camp that summer. It's something she remembers and cherishes too. For me, that exemplifies the love and the circle of friends that camp provides.

In November 2013, our daughter, Avalynn, was born. I think God knew we needed a reboot. Her name is a Celtic word meaning "wished for, prayed for, longed for child." Then in September 2015, we had a third son, Gabriel.

Growing up as a kid fighting and conquering cancer and then having friends who did not make it, I learned from a very young age how to live my life like it really means something, each and every day. As for the camp family, summer camp and the Christmas party

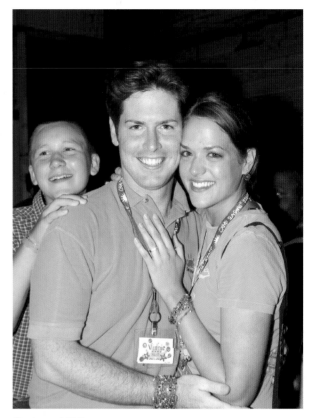

Kevin and Kelly

might be the only two times a year I see everyone, but as the years go by, these people have become my greatest friends.

Sometimes at camp kids resist when you ask them to put away their cell phones and iPads for a week (Camp Sunshine is device free). They think they can't do it. But I tell them, "Trust me, give it a week to be without those things and truly engage with other campers and the people beside you. Live your life versus chronicling your life on a social network. You are there to enjoy the moment. Try it." For example, to see a kid who does not know how to swim and who faces enormous physical challenges go home with a green bracelet because he passed the swim test . . . well, that's a feeling that's hard to beat.

For Kelly and me, cancer has been a part of our lives. I've beaten it twice, and she beat it herself. We're two star-crossed lovers, and cancer brought us together and allowed our story to happen. It's hard to be mad about that. Kelly's mother is now fighting acute myeloid leukemia. Maybe God put me through my adult leukemia so that we know how to best be there for her. Maybe I was the training program.

Camp is not just a place for kids with cancer to go and have fun—though it is definitely all that. It is a resource for the entire family because childhood cancer is a family disease—the entire family is struck. Camp Sunshine was the resource before anyone even knew there could be resources for families facing childhood cancer. Yes, in the early days of camp, there was some trial and error. But out of trial and error came knowledge, and that knowledge is unmatched. Consistently through the years, camp has created the programs that families need in times of crisis.

Camp is a lot more than a network and a resource, though. It becomes a huge family. That's what makes camp, camp.

JOHN AND CARLENE

Our journey to Camp Sunshine starts with the story of our daughter, Alicia. Alicia was diagnosed with AML, acute myeloid leukemia. When she was being treated for her cancer in 1984 and 1985, we learned about a camp that was started for kids with cancer, Camp Sunshine. Alicia didn't really want to go; we sort of pushed her into it. As a sixteen-year-old girl who was fighting cancer, she just felt so different from all the other kids she knew. Alicia was an only child. We thought camp and being around other kids who were fighting the same challenges she was would be good for her.

Alicia was incapacitated and in a wheelchair by the time she went to camp. Her legs weren't functioning by then. The ground at camp was so hilly that it was hard for her to get around in her wheelchair, so she made it her goal to walk some—and she did. For Alicia, this was a big accomplishment, and it was! When she came home at the end of the week, she was singing silly songs and telling us all kinds of stories. As her parents, it was hard to let her go to camp, but I can tell you we are so grateful we did.

Camp administrators emphasized that to help the campers get adjusted, they recommend that you not call your child and that they do not call you. When Alicia went to camp, we went to Cumberland Island. We forced ourselves to be away. When the day came for us to pick her up at camp, our Volkswagen broke down. We thought, "This is not a good day."

We made arrangements for one of the camp nurses to bring Alicia home. We were so upset that we wouldn't be there to pick her up and that somebody else was going to have to bring our daughter home, but Alicia didn't mind a bit. As an only child, she was as comfortable around adults as she was around kids her own age. I think she made friends with everybody at camp that week. It didn't bother her a bit that she had to go home with one of the nurses. That just

meant she could have some extra time with somebody from Camp Sunshine!

At first, we were all clueless that Alicia had cancer. In fact, right before her diagnosis, we took a week-long backpacking trip as a family. We also went whitewater rafting. We were a very active family; we loved the outdoors. We lived in Virginia Highlands, an in-town Atlanta neighborhood, and Alicia went to Grady High School in the city. But she liked hiking and nature. She had fun being out in the woods, and she loved climbing trees. That was part of who she was.

Once Alicia was diagnosed, it went quickly, and it wasn't long before she passed away. Afterward, we got involved in a grief group that Camp Sunshine sponsored. We met Tricia Benson there. Tricia talked with us about getting involved with camp as volunteers. Both John and I wanted to give back to that caring group of people and be involved with an organization that meant so much to Alicia and to us. We felt very privileged when they accepted us as volunteers. That summer turned into many, many years of volunteering at camp and Camp Sunshine becoming a big part of our lives.

We were angry when we lost Alicia, which is part of the process of losing a child. It is so frustrating to see your child go through this disease, knowing that she is so sick and there is nothing you can do about it. You

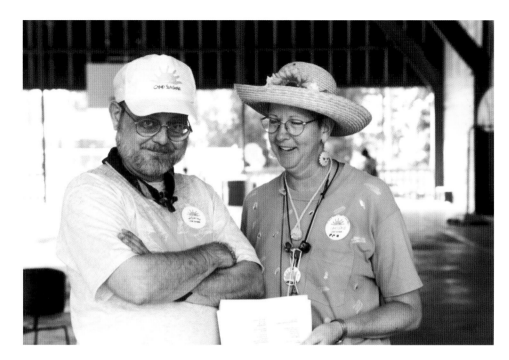

John and Carlene, camp counselors

live every day; you get through every day, one day at a time. It is all you can do. Then when parents lose their children, it puts such a strain on the marriage, and so often the marriage can be in trouble. Camp Sunshine gave us a common goal and a common ground, and we didn't grow apart, we didn't break up.

We left Atlanta about twelve years ago and now live in Port St. Joseph, Florida. But even after we left Atlanta, we came back to Georgia for a couple of years for summer camp. We just couldn't give it up. Going to camp has been a wonderful way for us to honor Alicia's memory. It meant a lot to us and we weren't ready to let it go.

Volunteering is an extremely hard job, especially as you get older. Every year when we got home from camp week, we were so exhausted that we slept for a day and a half! But it was worth every minute. Even though it is physically and mentally demanding, camp is incredible. We can't describe the satisfaction we felt knowing we had done something good for these children. Volunteers don't go to camp because they're looking for that reward, though; it's just the way it is at camp. The volunteers get as much out of the experience as the kids, maybe even more.

So even after twenty-seven or twenty-eight years, it was very hard for us to leave it all behind. At dinnertime, we still sometimes stand up and sing the Camp Sunshine dinner song (from Disney's *The Legend Of Johnny Appleseed*): "Oooooh, the Lord is good to me, and so I thank the Lord, for giving me the things I need, the sun and the rain and the apple seed. The Lord is good to me. Amen." Camp is just part of our lives, and we miss it very much.

We first met Kevin "Vinnie" Skelly when he was a seven-year-old camper and in John's cabin. Vinnie was having a hard time with some of his disease symptoms. Because he was not feeling physically well, he would wander off and not hang close to anybody else at first. He kept to himself a bit. From a seven-year-old's perspective, camp could be both exciting and scary. For Vinnie, and many of his cabinmates, camp was the first time away from home. Our job at camp was to make sure the boys had

an awesome time in a safe environment. By creating "Cabin Twenty-Three," the boys were no longer alone but were part of the Cabin Twenty-Three team. Every event, every meal, every polar bear swim was a team event. Before we knew it, Vinnie was having a great time with the other kids. For that week at camp, Vinnie and the other kids were treated just like normal kids, and that's the magic of camp. That's what Vinnie, like so many others, needed and appreciated.

Even when the campers are little, you can almost pick out who will go on to become counselors. They are the kids who "get with the program" and throw themselves into camp. They are the ones who get it. It was a joy to see Vinnie grow and mature every year. We were so proud when Vinnie returned to Camp Sunshine as a counselor. That meant a lot to us, and we knew he would be a great counselor.

We were always fond of Vinnie and grateful for his help at camp. Even as a very young camper, he would give up his rest period to help Carlene with the tie-dyeing. That first year, Carlene needed a place to set up the tie-dye station, so she had a kind of lean-to tent outside the arts and crafts building. Well, the lean-to fell apart the first time it rained—and we had a lot of rain that summer! Getting a better tent helped, but things would still get crazy in there! Tie-dyeing would stay open during rest period so the adults could come get their tie-dyeing done too. They dyed everything: their underwear, their T-shirts, their tops. Everybody loved it. Vinnie would rinse out the clothes that had been tie-dyed, and if you've ever done tie-dyeing, you know that's a big and physical job.

Tie-dying is how Vinnie met his wife, Kelly. We love that story, and we've been thinking a lot about that connection. We had no idea that the things we did when Vinnie was a young boy at camp would impact him even into adulthood. It was an honor for us to know we have had a positive impact on Vinnie. Of course, we didn't participate in camp for that reason; we just wanted to give the kids a break from the world of doctors and nurses and hospitals and treatment. We hope that's what we accomplished.

Some of the best moments at camp were spontaneous. One that was touching for us was a night when some of the adult volunteers went to Cracker Barrel for dinner—just for a little break—and everybody went around the room telling their story. We didn't have to, but everyone did. All the boo-hooing that went on that night! That dinner made us feel close to the other volunteers and created a special bond between us all. It was astounding to find so many good people in one

place, all working together with one purpose: to be there for these kids.

John had been in the marines, and when he first started heading up the boys' cabin, he ran it like the marines. He would have the boys marching in a row like little ducks, with John standing at the head of the line, and in the lunchroom, he would have the boys rhythmically bang on the tables. John wanted them to understand how important it was that they remain there for each other. He wanted to create a camaraderie that the kids were one cabin, one team, and one camp, that they all stayed together.

Camp Sunshine is a good thing in what can be a bad world. People have to do good to offset the bad. Kids at camp come from different socioeconomic backgrounds. These things might matter on the outside, but at camp they don't make a difference. The kids are encouraged to comingle into one cohesive group, and suddenly instead of being the kid with cancer, they are part of a group of friends, and it just so happens that all of them have cancer. They're not different anymore. Camp is special because the kids learn that cancer happens to other kids and other families, too, and that they are not alone in this.

Vinnie and Kelly Skelly are an amazing family. It's incredible all the things they have done, especially when you understand all that they have been through together. It is an honor to be part of Vinnie's story.

JANE

I remember Vinnie as a seven-year-old coming to camp for the first time. He was little when I first knew him, and he was always in the middle of things in that little boy cabin! It wasn't until his son Everett died that I wrote him a little note. I got a note right back from him. Each year on the anniversary of Everett's death, I drop Vinnie a note to say that I'm thinking about him.

When Vinnie was diagnosed a second time, he called to tell me about his recurrence. He called me because he knew I worked with adults that had cancer. We had a relationship, and he trusted my advice. He got to a doctor that was really good. I encouraged him to stay there and not wander around. I was really glad to see him when he came back to camp after his treatment.

I like Vinnie's resilience. He and Kelly have a strong faith that helps them get through the challenges they have had to face at a young age. They seem to move along through what life has dealt them.

Vinnie's thoughtful, kind, and compassionate. He came back to camp last year as a counselor and I got to see him in action a lot. You can tell that he's engaged in his campers' experience.

I believe if you can be helpful and supportive in a small way, it is important to do what you can for people that are a part of your family or "tribe." If life is hard for them, I want to do what little things I can to hopefully lift them up a little bit. If things are good, I still do the same thing.

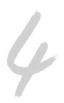

A special girl in Cabin Nine

Kelly Skelly (born January 16, 1981; hometown: Marietta, Georgia)
and Nanci "Bubbles" Dubin

KELLY

It was the summer of 1995. I was in marching band as a freshman in high school, and during these exercises, I could tell something was going on in my neck. Something wasn't right. At first, I ignored it. I was fifteen years old at the time. One night after band practice, I came home and talked to my mom about it. We went to my room, and I lay down on the bed. My mom started feeling around my neck and said she felt something swollen.

The next day my mom took me straight to my primary care doctor. He did a blood test, but it came back and showed nothing. Initially, my parents thought it might be mono. There was a lot of mono going around. My sister had had it, and a lot of kids in school had it. But my parents weren't satisfied. They said, "No, we'd

like further testing. What else can we do to find out what this is?"

Soon thereafter, a biopsy was done. They took a lymph node out. It took several days to get the results back. But the biopsy showed that I had cancer. I remember the doctor called us after hours, like 7:00 p.m., so I knew something was really wrong. But I was in la-la-land as a teenager, right? I didn't know anything about cancer. I remember he was teary eyed when we walked into his office the next day. In the same sentence, he told us that this was cancer and that I would see an oncologist, Dr. Steve Lauer at Egleston Hospital. Within a couple of days, I was sitting at Egleston and learning about Hodgkin's lymphoma. The doctors were already getting together a treatment protocol and had already scheduled a port (port-a-cath) to be inserted for my first chemotherapy. Things were moving so quickly; it was bam, bam, bam!

The cancer was in my neck and my upper chest. If it had been in my lower chest, they would have had to do radiation. As it was, I avoided all of that because the cancer was caught so quickly. It was truly a miracle. It was also a life lesson in being persistent and advocating for my own health. I learned that you can't necessarily take one doctor's word for it. It is OK, and it is important, to get second opinions.

I remember my medical team telling me, "If you're going to have cancer, this is the one to have." They discussed favorable cure rates and outcomes with me. That soothed my parents at least. But I was young, and when I heard the word cancer, I assumed I was going to die. I had a lot to learn about this disease. I didn't know any young people at that time who had cancer. I had no clue what any of this meant.

The summer of '96 was my first Camp Sunshine camp. I didn't even know there was a camp like this for kids with cancer. I had awesome nurses in the hospital who kept telling me, "You've got to go to camp, you've got to go." But I thought, *Yeah, right, a camp with a bunch of depressed people who are in wheelchairs and dying of cancer?* Honestly, that's what I thought.

When you are young, a teenager with cancer, there is so much you have to deal with. I knew students at school who thought they would catch this from me. They didn't know; they needed to be educated and informed, too, but I didn't want to be the girl with cancer. I didn't want to go to camp. If anything, I wanted to distance myself from other people who would give me that stigma. I just wanted to be a teenager again. I wanted to look forward to things, to not dwell on cancer and everything that had happened to me. In the end, my parents made me go.

Most teenagers don't want to feel limited. They don't want people to feel sorry for them. And they don't want anyone to know they have this disease. Those are all reasons kids might resist the idea of camp. But camp was exactly the opposite of what I was thinking it would be. My very first day at Camp Sunshine, my eyes were opened to a whole new way of looking at things. I slid into the pace of camp right away. I pretty much did everything, every activity camp offered. I never did the same activity more than once until I had gone through the entire list. I literally tried everything.

It's funny how God orchestrates things, how He provides. Bubbles and Kim were my counselors in Cabin Nine, and those two counselors alone made a night and

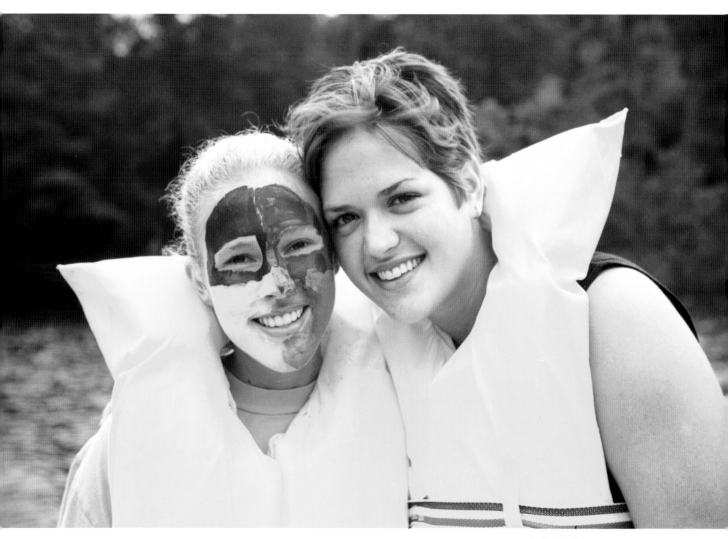

Kelly (right), summer camp

day difference in my attitude. Bubbles left a great impression on me. From my very first day at camp, she instilled certain things in me: there would be no comparing ourselves to others, and there would be no self-doubts. We were there to have fun. Bubbles helped lift that load for a first-time camper, especially one like me who wasn't sure she even wanted to be there. Bubbles has been there for me ever since.

And then there were my cabinmates! Within eight hours I had made instant friends with the girls in my cabin. Two of the girls had the same diagnosis as me. I went from not knowing anyone with cancer to knowing two girls my age with the exact same disease.

Even more life changing, I met a camper named Kevin "Vinnie" Skelly. Kevin's earliest memory of me is seeing me in an arts and crafts class. I was making a dream catcher. My first memory of him was at the ice cream social. I remember seeing a group of guys and assuming this one guy was maybe a counselor. He looked a little older, he was well dressed and talking maturely, and he seemed almost like a celebrity. I just remember I didn't want anything to do with him. I didn't go to camp looking for a boyfriend.

The next day, a letter appeared in the "Dear Gabby" gossip column in the daily camp newsletter asking, "Who's the special girl in Cabin Nine?" Everyone was

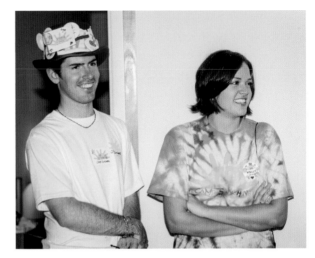

Kevin and Kelly

buzzing about it . . . Who could this be? Who's writing this? Who is he asking about? At the talent show, Kevin sang a song, "Only Wanna Be with You" by Hootie and the Blowfish, and he said, "This goes out to a special girl in Cabin Nine." I turned red as a beet. I was so embarrassed.

Kevin persisted in pursuing me, and by the end of the week, we had grown fond of each other. We had cabin porch time at night, and we had started chitchatting with each other. He let me know he was leaving camp on Friday, a day early, for a choir trip. So before he left, he found me at the pool and said, "I just want to say goodbye." Then he pulled me toward him and kissed me on the cheek. A lot of letters went back and forth between us after that first camp. What a lost thing that is in our current culture—writing letters, actual letters, to each other!

But when I came home, I didn't want the focus to be, "Hey, I met this guy." Being at camp was a special time, and I wanted to hold onto that. Yes, the relationship and the attention from Kevin did make me feel very special. But we were two years apart in age, and I wasn't sure what would happen next or where it would be going.

After that first summer camp, I made sure I didn't miss a single camp program. I participated in teen retreats, an outdoor adventure trip, and a trip to Washington, D.C. Literally every program I could get to, I was there. I was blessed to get to go to those activities, and they strengthened my bond with Camp Sunshine even more. When I graduated from camp after my senior year in high school, I immediately enrolled as a counselor in training, and when I was twenty-one, I began my tenure as a volunteer camp counselor. For years, I did not miss a summer at camp.

Kevin proposed to me during the summer of 2005 at camp, on the grassy knoll where I first saw him.

We were married in May 2006. We asked two of our best Camp Sunshine friends, Christopher Thurman and Bubbles, to be our ring bearer and flower girl. Our Camp Sunshine friends are just incredible and a lot of them—Sally Hale, Brinsley Thigpen, Emily Garner, Kati Tanner Gardner, Sara Woznicki—were at our wedding. Kevin and I always say we have multiple families: our *family*, our church family, and our Camp Sunshine family.

As cancer survivors, the number one topic we are all worried about is marriage and children. Whether or not you can have children—we all share that same concern. There is no way you can test for that, so there is no way to know ahead of time. Kevin was set on having two children, but me, I wanted five! Still, we wouldn't know if we could have children until we started trying. My sister said, "Kelly, the thing is, you can believe some of what the doctors are saying, but you don't have to accept all of it as absolute truth. God knows the desires of your heart, and He will answer your prayers."

Within the first months of trying to conceive, we learned we were expecting, and on August 3, 2010, our first child, our son Liam, was born. I had to miss camp that summer for the first time. When they placed him in my arms, my whole world changed.

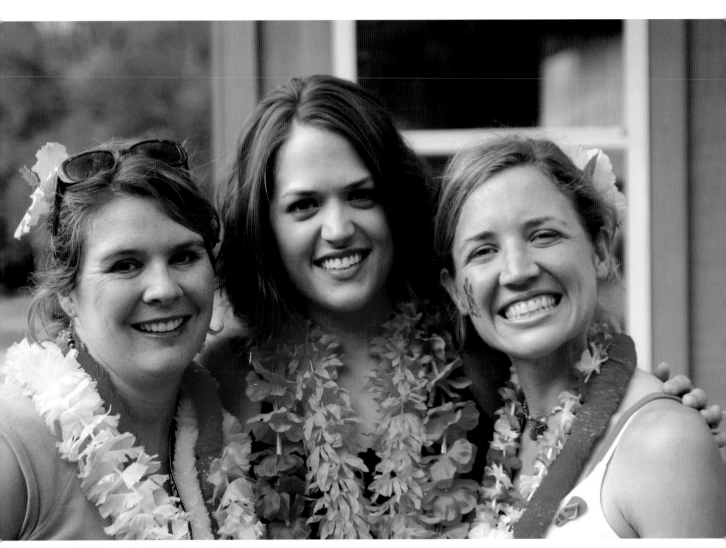

Kelly (center) with fellow counselors

In April 2012, our second son, Everett, was born. When Everett passed away unexpectedly three months later, everything changed. I went from being a free-spirited kind of mom, not a helicopter parent at all, to being a complete nervous wreck. Kevin and I kept Liam on a heart monitor for ten months following his brother's death just for the peace of mind—just to be able to sleep at night.

A few years later, in 2016, our family faced another challenge. Something started changing with Kevin's health. I noticed he was tired, fatigued, and he'd come home from work with bruises on his arms. He'd tell me he was tired, but I thought, *I'm tired too.* I didn't know he was feeling as badly as he was.

About that time, I had flown to Miami for a cruise. The day before boarding, Kevin called me. He had gone in for blood work. His blood counts were completely off. He kept saying, "Don't worry about me. I'll be fine." He wanted me to go on the trip, but he also told me his doctor said he needed to go to the ER. Within a couple of hours, we learned that his platelets had dropped to seven thousand; they're supposed to be one hundred thousand. He had no energy at all. I knew I couldn't get on that ship. I flew back to Atlanta as soon as possible and headed straight to the ER. When Kevin saw me

and started walking toward me, he collapsed. I somehow got him back in the bed and called the nurses.

Fortunately, the doctor on call in the ER happened to be a hematologist-oncologist, who ordered an MRI and CT scan. He also ordered a bone marrow biopsy. The pathology report indicated acute lymphoblastic leukemia, the same disease as Kevin's first diagnosis. We were sent straight to Northside Hospital, where Kevin repeated every test and went straight from diagnosis to treatment.

Kevin's sister was a perfect match for the bone marrow transplant, which was his best chance at remission. Again, a miracle in our lives.

There were multiple times that year when we didn't know what the outcome would be. There were travel restrictions and restrictions on being in public due to Kevin's high risk of infection. For the first time in decades, Kevin had to miss summer camp. But it strengthened us even more. Through it all, we came out fighting. Again. We reached a point where we hit rock bottom, but we learned to take it step by step and walk through it one step at a time.

Kevin and I both say it was no fun getting a cancer diagnosis, not at all. Nobody wants that for their child or for anyone they love. But we also see the blessings in it. We realize we wouldn't have met each other, we wouldn't have had these friends, we wouldn't have known all these wonderful people, we wouldn't have the life we have had. I know that some people might not understand, but I look at my diagnosis as a blessing.

People ask me, how can you go through so much? God provides. And one of the ways He provides is by giving us family and the friends we need. Our camp family is enormously encouraging and uplifting and always has been. My goal is to get back to camp, when Kevin and I are back on our feet again. And we will be back.

NANCI ("BUBBLES")

All of the days I've spent in the children's hospital and at camp, witnessing firsthand what these children with cancer go through, has completely changed my perspective on things. I know the strength of these children.

Kelly was a specific case in point. I love Kelly. I always called her "Kelly Belly," and when she married Kevin, I could call her "Kelly Belly Skelly." I had her as a camper when she was a teenager. She was going through chemotherapy, like so many of the kids, but for some reason, she never lost her hair. We used to think it was because the hospital gave her this crazy cap, like a double heating pad, to wear on her head. Everybody else was bald and Kelly wasn't, but she always had this incredible empathy for everyone around her.

Kelly and I go way back to the days when campers sat on their counselors' beds and talked to them or lay on their backs and looked at the ceiling and just talked and talked. That's what Kelly would do. I remember her telling me once, "You're like a second mom to me." I am so honored that she feels that way. When Kelly graduated from camp and became a volunteer counselor herself, it was like we had come full circle.

There's a mutual appreciation we have for each other . . . one that started with Camp Sunshine. We both lead busy lives now, and we have both had a lot happen to us. Through the years, we have never let the bond between us be broken. I have been a support system for Kelly, and she has been one for me. When she and Kevin got married, I was honored to be the flower girl at their wedding. When Kevin was diagnosed with his second cancer, I sent him an email every day for a year. I wanted them both to know I was there for them, just as they would be there for me. When Kelly and Kevin lost a child, it was like it had happened to my own family member. That's just how deep the ties are.

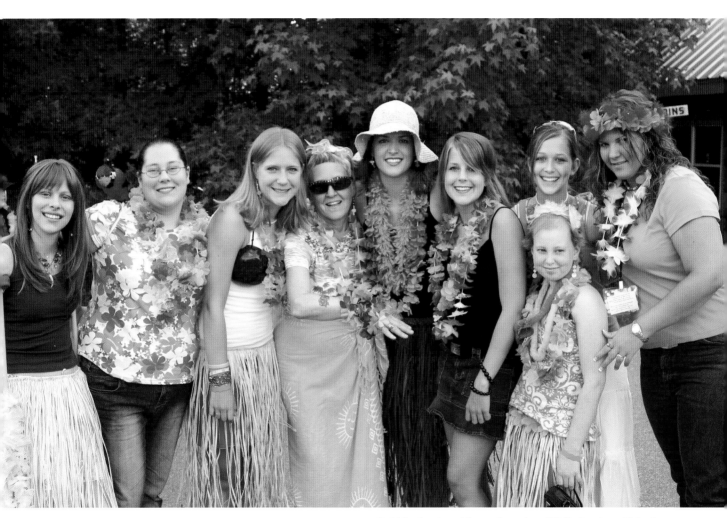

Bubbles (center with sunglasses) and Kelly (center with hat)

I lost my mother to cancer at a very young age. I have no children of my own. I didn't go as a camp volunteer to find a family. I was a schoolteacher for years, and when I stopped teaching, I missed the children. At camp, I've met the most remarkable children, the most remarkable people anyone would ever want to meet. Camp has given me a family.

When a lot of people reach my age, their motto unfortunately is *no, no, no, no*. But mine is *go, try, be, do*. It is because of Camp Sunshine that I have this attitude. There is no stopping the connections we make at camp. There is no end to the love and dedication and bonds made there.

We're all the same

Sakarrai Sanders (born May 23, 1987; hometown: Hinesville, Georgia) and Stephanie Lewis Gibson

SAKARRAI

I was diagnosed with acute lymphocytic leukemia (ALL) in 1992, treated with chemotherapy for two years, and went into remission in 1994. That was my first year at Camp Sunshine.

It was second grade and I was seven years old. I was living in Hinesville, Georgia, where my dad was stationed at Fort Stewart-Hunter Army Airfield. I don't remember my diagnosis too well, but my dad told me that I asked to be picked up all the time. I was four years old, and he thought it was because I didn't want to walk. He would say, "No, you're fine. You can walk." Then he realized there was a problem when I started crying, and that's when he took me to the doctor, and I received a diagnosis of arthritis. He thought, *There's no way a four-year-old could have arthritis*. He requested a

second opinion from a military doctor, an oncologist, and that's when my parents discovered I had ALL. I was diagnosed in June 1992, right after I turned five.

The diagnosis was really hard on my dad and my mom. I remember my mom sitting on the bed crying; she just wouldn't stop crying. I still get a little emotional thinking about it because I've only seen my mom cry three times and that was the first time. I wondered, "What's wrong? It's OK. It's fine." I don't think I understood the effect of cancer, what could have happened if it wasn't caught early or if they didn't treat it. I didn't understand.

I remember losing my hair and not thinking much about it. I was at the Ronald McDonald House (which houses families of children during treatment and long stays at the local children's hospital) with my dad. He had just combed my hair while I played with this hot

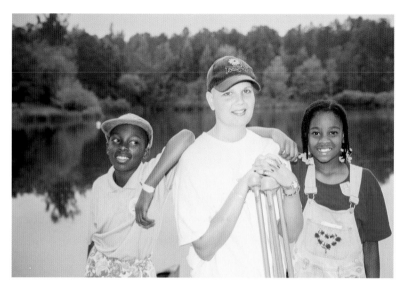

Sakarrai (right) with fellow campers

pink Barbie convertible doll and my hair started coming out. It was curly then, and it dropped on the floor. I recall saying, "Here you go, Daddy." He just went quiet and put the hair in a Ziploc bag. We still have it to this day.

It feels like it was such a long time ago. I think my cancer diagnosis was extremely hard on my parents, more than I could imagine. I just know it was, after seeing my mom cry. I went to Texas for a little bit, to Brooke Army Medical Center, to get treated. My dad was in Texas as a compassionate reassignment because the army had really good medical professionals in San Antonio, and my mom was in Georgia. I remember when I left to go back to Georgia, he started crying. I thought he was crying because he had bumped his head putting me on the airplane because the ceilings are kind of low—that's what he said. Now I know, he was crying because I was leaving.

My treatment lasted for two years, and I went into remission when I was seven. I went to Camp Sunshine for the first time that year. I remember I didn't want to go to camp. I was shy and nervous; I was an only child at the time and didn't want to be away from my parents. They told me that I had to go. My dad said, "You are going to this camp." My parents drove me all the way up to camp, and I cried when they dropped me off. I remember meeting Sally, Dorothy, Jane, and, of course, my counselors Tricia and Verwray. Then I just felt at home. I was so nervous at the beginning of the week, but by the end, I didn't want to go home. I cried when my parents came to pick me up from camp!

One of my best memories from that first year of camp was the "mix-match" dance. We all wore silly mismatched clothes! Christina, a cabinmate, and I switched clothes. A picture from that year shows me with Christina, and I'm wearing one of her pink Keds, one of my white sneakers, red striped shorts, blue T-shirt, and face paint and have my arms wrapped adoringly around our counselor.

I loved fishing. Jane, the fishing activity counselor that year, has a lot of pictures of me fishing and holding up fish. I remember catching my first fish—my first time fishing ever! Another favorite activity was gold panning. The gold-panning activity was tucked up into the woods with a perfect view of the lake. The sluices were stocked with fool's gold and what we thought were real gems! A counselor made the rounds to department stores earlier in the year to get costume jewelry donated and the staff "spiked" the sand with these precious gems. I also loved archery, and we even had skeet shooting. The FBI ran the skeet-shooting activity for Camp Sunshine. That was one of my favorites—it was so cool!

For seven years, I went to camp. My first year was in 1994, and my last year as a camper was 2001 because my family moved to Missouri in 2002 when my dad got stationed at Fort Leonard Wood. If my family hadn't moved, I would have still gone to camp. That was one of the hardest times of my life when we moved.

Another fond memory of all those times at camp is the block party. It's like an impromptu street party! At least impromptu to the campers—because I know now that it's planned by the staff to feel that way. Stephanie Lewis, now Gibson, Natasha, and I used to go together. We would just walk around being super cute, trying to act older than we were, and look at guys. Even getting up early to go polar bear swim (early morning swim time before breakfast) with my camp buddies was fun.

Looking back, I have sad memories too. There was a camper, Reggie, who passed away when he was fourteen. He asked me during junior week to go to the dance with him, but I wanted to go with another guy. This is

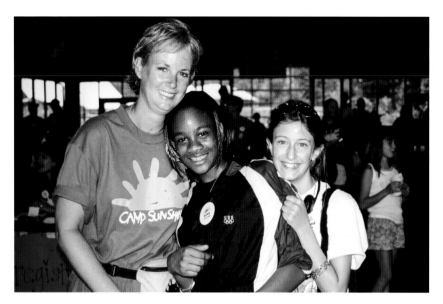

Sakarrai (center) with counselor and camper Stephanie

so terrible to remember, but I told him no. When he saw me at the dance with the other guy, he cried in the gym in the corner. I felt so bad. He was from Savannah, too, so when we all rode the bus back, I talked to him and I tried to cheer him up because he was really sad about it. We did stay in touch. He had a relapse and had to get a bone marrow transplant, which did not go well. Soon after his bone marrow transplant, he passed away. I went to his funeral, and it was so sad, and I still remember how I felt today.

My family and I went to the Savannah family camp (a Camp Sunshine family camp) two times. I remember Jane Clark the most out of any of the staff there. We brought my cousin and little sister, who was maybe a year and a half or two, with us. She was really little. Even though it was a short weekend, it was a blast. I remember we made a chocolate lollipop mold in a cooking class. I thought that was really cool. I can't remember too much else, but I know I had a good time and that it was good for my family, to see that we weren't the only ones around that had a kid with cancer. I'm glad that my family got to experience a part of Camp Sunshine.

I went to college on an ROTC scholarship at Lincoln University in Jefferson City, Missouri. I needed a waiver to join ROTC because I had cancer, and I did not know how that was going to unfold. The army is particular about being in "good health." My dad was a recruiter, and he said, "They're probably not going to accept you because you've had cancer." I told him, "Well, I'm going to try anyway." I saw a few doctors, and none of them felt comfortable completing the paperwork to give me clearance. I then reached out to my oncologist, Col. James Barker, since he had followed me and provided my healthcare ever since I went into remission. He wrote the letter to the military documenting my well-being. I received my waiver and was accepted, and it all worked out. I felt like getting the waiver was another sign from God, telling me I should join the military.

Last year, (Camp Sunshine volunteer) Mo asked me, "What do you do?" I told him, "I'm in the army." After sharing that with Mo, several kids approached me asking questions and saying, "I didn't know you could join the army if you've had cancer!" I happily told them, "Yes, you can."

Camp Sunshine means acceptance. When I was a camper, a counselor told me, "Don't change who you are." She said that I had such a cheerful spirit and advised "don't ever change that." I take that with me now, from age seven. I'm thirty-one, and it's still with me.

At camp you don't have to worry about being judged. Every year that I was at camp, the counselors always welcomed me with open arms and embraced me and who I was. They genuinely care about you. You can sense that. They take the time to get to know you. I think that acceptance is what camp is all about. Camp Sunshine taught me to be a confident person. I don't think I would be the same person that I am today without camp.

In the time since I attended camp, I've reconnected with Stephanie Gibson. We were in the same cabin for a few years, and she was part of my Camp Sunshine journey. I was so happy once she sought me out years after camp.

Stephanie and I were close. She meant a lot to me—we had a special connection since both of us were from Savannah and rode the Savannah bus to camp together. We went polar bear swimming early each day and would do all camp activities together. I love Stephanie, and I loved being with her and my cabinmates Michelle and Natasha. They all mean a lot to me.

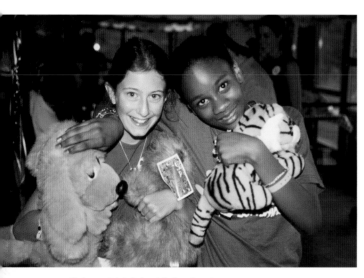

Sakarrai (right) with Stephanie

I always look forward to going to Camp Sunshine and volunteering. I see it as a way of giving back. So much was poured into me, and I want to be able to do the same for campers today and maybe help them become more confident because life can be hard. Life's tough. I feel like you need solid values to deal with life's challenges. When that counselor said, "Don't ever change who you are. You're beautiful just the way you are," that helped me more than I can begin to say. Today a lot of kids have low self-esteem and Camp Sunshine helps build kids up. Camp not only helps them deal with cancer but helps them become better people. Then maybe campers can pass it along too.

Camp is like a lifeline that is always there. I feel like it's a part of me since the day I arrived when I was seven. I have always had Camp Sunshine in my heart. It's just the way that you are treated, not only as a camper but also as a counselor. It's like family. It's pure happiness, pure sunshine.

Having cancer made me a better person. I'm much more grateful. Being at camp makes me see things in a different light, and I am very fortunate to be a part of this community.

Camp Sunshine's biggest takeaway for me is that we're all equal. Everybody's the same here. You do not get that anywhere else in society. Camp is the one place where everybody is the same, regardless of gender or race. You are accepted just as you are. *We're all the same.*

STEPHANIE

Sakarrai is one of those people you meet in life and you never, ever forget. We met in 1995 at Camp Sunshine and had an immediate connection.

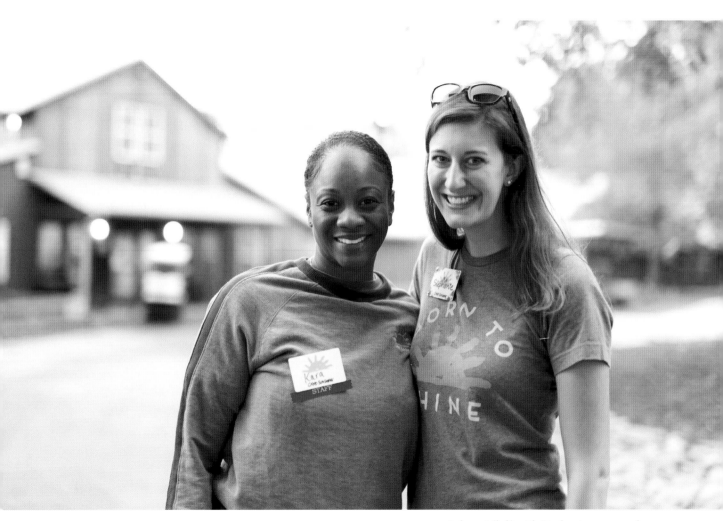

Sakarrai (left) with Stephanie, as counselors

We both lived a long way from camp, so we rode the Savannah bus to get there every year. Once we arrived at camp, we stayed in the same cabin, too, so that's a lot of time to be together and get to know each other. It's a long drive from Savannah to camp. Asking your parents to drive you there and then come back and pick you up, that's a lot to expect. So for us, the bus was a great option. It was just so much fun—a part of the whole camp experience for us. Usually a nurse or a parent would ride over with us and lots and lots of good friends, like Michelle and Natasha. We would talk and laugh all the way to camp and then sleep all the way home to Savannah after camp. We'd be exhausted!

I love that Sakarrai and I were both from the Savannah area and had that bond of not just having cancer but the shared experience of getting to and from camp and being cabinmates. As we aged out of camp, we lost touch with each other for a while. But then I began "stalking" her on Facebook, and when we finally connected, we picked up exactly where we had left off. And the years apart? We've covered all that and tied it all up with a bow, and now, we're keeping the connection strong.

6

A hidden treasure

Stephanie Lewis Gibson, MD (born January 5, 1987; hometown: Savannah, Georgia), and Jane Clark

STEPHANIE

I was very young—an infant—so I don't remember my surgery and treatment. I've learned details of my cancer diagnosis from my parents and doctors over the years. I was eighteen months old when I was diagnosed with Wilms tumor, stage 2, which basically is a rare kidney cancer that affects children. I know there was a huge mass associated with it, and I know I was part of a fifteen-month clinical trial to get rid of the cancer. Today the standard of care takes six months, but regrettably, that shorter course of treatment didn't exist when I was diagnosed. Fortunately, I did very well and went into remission. My last chemotherapy was on October 25, 1989, and I have remained cancer-free ever since.

I grew up in the Savannah area. Treatment for childhood cancer was not available in Savannah back in the 1980s, so my parents had to drive me to Augusta weekly for my treatments. Although I was far away from Atlanta and camp, I was able to make the connection. My first summer at camp was in 1995, when I was eight years old.

One of my clearest memories of camp is skeet shooting. I remember waking up in the morning and hearing gunshots, but it was just campers doing skeet shooting. Another memory is swimming in the lake, which was so much fun. I also remember one time there was an elaborate prank where somebody from "the FBI" showed up and "kidnapped" Sally Hale. That was a lot of fun. I used to love the camper-counselor challenges too. I'm competitive by nature, so I really enjoyed those.

When I was older, I joined the high school trip to Washington, D.C. I loved that trip. My favorite part

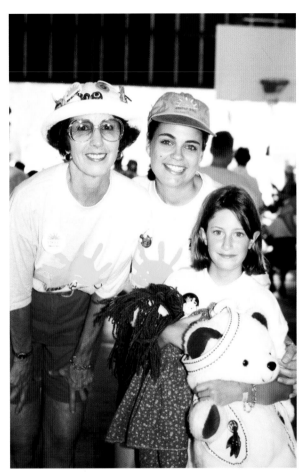

Stephanie at junior camp with counselors

was going to the FBI Training Academy. It was such a neat thing for a young person to do. No one else, none of my other friends from outside of camp, got to do that when they went to Washington. But we did! We also got to lay a wreath at the Tomb of the Unknown Soldier. That was very moving and an incredible honor.

My experience at Camp Sunshine helped shape and guide my decision to become a pediatrician. I liked science and was very much a science nerd, but there wasn't one particular point in my life where I decided, *Yes, I want to be a doctor.* There wasn't an "aha" moment. Growing up at camp, I was around a lot of medical providers: pediatricians, oncologists, and nurses. Even though I wasn't diagnosed and treated as an older child, I was around cancer and the medical world associated with it: the checkups, the follow-ups, camp, my friends who had cancer. I was definitely in the cancer world, and that world made sense to me. So the idea of doing something in medicine or becoming a doctor just fit and felt right for me.

I now practice as a pediatrician at Palmetto Health in Richland, South Carolina. My work is my passion. I love it. I love kids. I love how resilient they are. Take the kids at camp. They are getting hit with these unbelievable medical challenges and diagnoses, and they

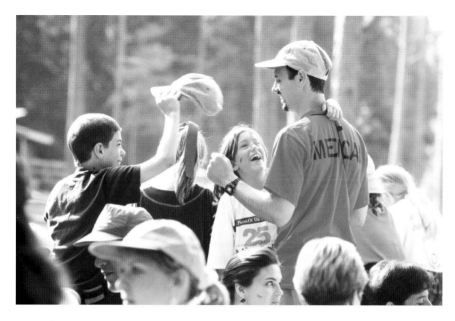

Stephanie (center) at junior camp

are super strong. They come out fighting. It is amazing how strong these kids are emotionally, physically, and in every other way.

One thing I have taken away from my camp experience and applied to my practice as a pediatrician is being mindful to talk to children at their level. I say things directly to them, like, "I hear you're sick. Tell me what's going on." I've learned how important it is to describe things—especially medical things—to kids so that they understand more fully what's going on. I try hard to avoid talking over them or talking only to their parents. Kids can be scared and sad when they are sick, and it is best to talk with them at a level they can understand.

I had to take a break from my camp volunteer duties to pursue my medical degree. I felt a terrible loss those years, like I was missing out. It was a huge gap in my life to go without Camp Sunshine. When I returned to camp as a cabin counselor in 2013, I was placed in a cabin with Jane Clark. We hit it off right away. We balance each other very well, and we're now a well-oiled machine!

My husband is extremely supportive of my commitment to camp. He knows the week of camp is protected time for me. Nothing touches camp week. He is in my corner about that and defends my time at camp against all distractions. He gets how very important camp is to me. When we got married, we even set the date in July to deliberately fall after summer camp week. My husband might not follow the motions and sing along to "Wagon Wheel" (a popular camp song), but he does get camp and what it means to me.

It's hard to explain the Camp Sunshine experience. Honestly, I feel like these people are my family. They shaped who I am today and how I have developed as an adult. At camp, nobody makes fun of you. No one judges you. From the very beginning, everyone was so genuinely friendly and caring. People are truly so nice. Everyone is positive and accepts you just the way you are. How could anyone not love this? How could you not want this to be a big part of your life?

The focus at Camp Sunshine isn't that you're a kid with cancer and that's why you go to camp and that's what you want to talk about while you are there. In fact,

it's the opposite. Camp is about going to this amazing place with these amazing friends and doing these amazing activities. And *oh, by the way, everybody has cancer.*

Just recently, a girl in my cabin turned to another camper, who was bald, and asked, "Oh, did you lose your hair because you have cancer?" The camper responded, "Yes." Then the first girl said, "Oh, I have cancer too." Then another girl said, "So do I!" and then another and another said the same thing. It was like a huge realization for them. Finally, one girl said, "OK, raise your hand if you have cancer," and of course, everybody raised their hand. I raised my hand too. "Miss Stephanie, you have cancer too?" It can be a powerful thing to talk about your cancer experiences in a setting like that.

Being both a young camper and now an adult volunteer, I see the positive impact Camp Sunshine has on these kids, and it is awesome. Camp is so special that we are all careful and hesitant about who we recommend being a volunteer. The last thing we want is for someone to go for one year and then not go back. That's not what camp is about. Camp is about consistency and commitment from everyone. Even my brother knows that. My brother wanted to volunteer. But bringing my brother to camp to meet everyone was like bringing a

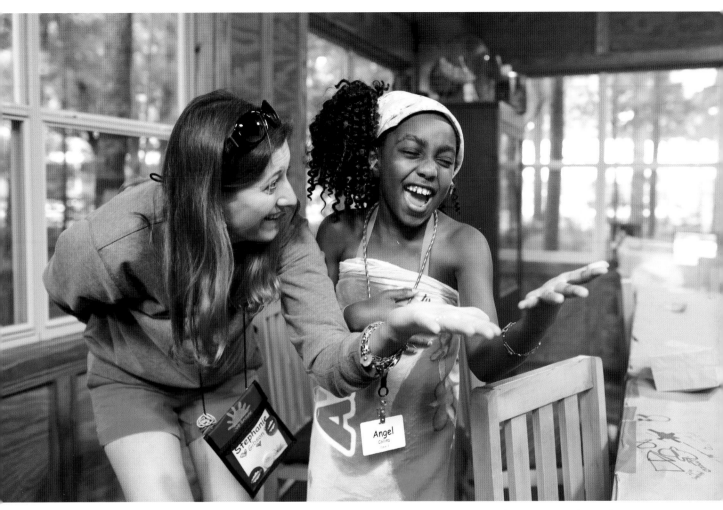

Stephanie as counselor with camper

date to meet my parents for the first time. It was nerve wracking! I am thrilled to say he did very well, though, and that he loves camp too. Camp is like a hidden treasure—and when you find it, you know it is a precious thing that you want to hold on to forever.

JANE

My commitment to oncology goes back to my brother, who was diagnosed with leukemia when he was fifteen. I was still in college, studying nursing at Emory University. My parents called me one night, and they told me what was wrong and asked me where they should take him. I got to make that decision. I remember that part. I asked them to bring him to Emory, so he was treated at Egleston Children's Hospital.

I had heard about the efforts to start camp from Sally Hale, and I said, "Yeah, I'd like to be involved if you ever get a chance to do that." I got involved the second year. Since then, I have been a cabin counselor to seven- to nine-year-old girls. To me, that is the best age group to work with at camp because everything is new. It's just the excitement that you see. Every three years, when I get a new group of girls, I get to see camp in a different way.

Recently, I had an opportunity to go to both junior camp and teen camp, which was just a delight for me because I got to see the kids that I've had from the beginning and how they've grown up and what they're getting ready to do. One of my cabins just graduated this past year. The girls are just so excited about what they're going to do. There are five of them that have been together for the whole twelve years of camp. It's just sweet. I love that.

From the beginning, I was ready for Camp Sunshine. In the early years of camp, it was rustic. We had screens on the sides of the cabins, and when it rained in the middle of the night, which it did often, we had to move all the beds to the center of the room in the middle of the night with kids still sleeping in them so they wouldn't get all wet.

Over the years, the facilities have changed. The number of people that we have coming and volunteering for long periods of time has changed. The rules have also changed a little bit, and we are a bigger organization. What has not changed is that kids all of a sudden find themselves here. I was looking at a kid this summer who was at camp for the first time. He was a teenager, and he stood around for the first hour and a half looking sort of gawky, but by the end of the day, he was singing "Kermit the Frog" (a favorite camp

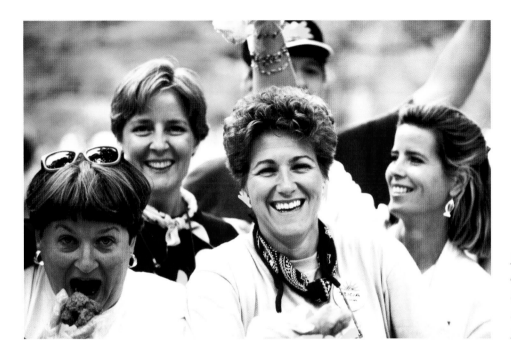

Jane (far left) with counselors Tricia (center), Dorothy (right), and Maggie Riley (back left)

song). In just six hours, the campers were all hugging and hanging on because people made that happen. It doesn't make any difference what history or disease you come with. Somebody's going to pay attention to you and is going to be your friend at Camp Sunshine.

When I try to explain Camp Sunshine to people, I always talk about the experience of leaving your immediate family. You will look for people who are your family in a different way. I consider myself to have had three families. One of them was my immediate family. The second one I found at my junior college. And the third family I was lucky enough to find was at camp. What makes us a family is common values. I do not think it matters how you think about things outside of camp. It's how you think about other people, how important they are, what they mean to you and your life, and hopefully what you mean to them and their lives. It's finding your tribe. It is who is important to you and how they help you be a better person. And hopefully, you help them be a better person too.

I learned a lot of life lessons at Camp Sunshine. Everyone does. One year, I had a camper who couldn't talk because of her radiation treatments. She had this tiny voice and couldn't move her tongue. We were doing a talent show. I thought of a skit for the girls. They would lie on their backs on a table and turn upside down, draw eyes on their chins, and put sheets around them, creating the illusion that they were right side up. The camper who had trouble talking couldn't hold her head upside down for long because it made her dizzy. We were trying to think of something for her to do. I said, "She's going to be the announcer." My cocounselors all looked at me and said, "That might not make sense for her to be the announcer—she can't talk very well." I said, "She's going to talk for this one. She doesn't have to say much. She'll be fine. She'll love to do it." I asked the camper, and she said, "Oh yeah, please, yes, I want to be our announcer." The night of the talent show, she got up there and said her lines using the microphone. The kids all sang a song upside down, and everybody was happy! She did it! When we had the kids draw pictures of their favorite camp experience, she drew a detailed picture of all the little girls hanging upside down and the counselors behind them holding their legs so they wouldn't fall off the table and showed herself with a microphone off to the side with her whole speech in a bubble. There are these little teeny moments like that when you know you're doing the right thing.

One of my other favorite camp stories is of another little camper, of her daddy carrying her in. She was seven. I had seen them at family camp. The daddy never put the child down. I had never seen her feet touch the ground. She was still on treatment. He carried her into camp. I thought, well, I am not carrying this child all week. That's not going to work. I don't believe she had gotten dirt on the bottom of her shoes since she'd been diagnosed. When her dad came to pick her up, she ran to him. He tried to pick her up, and she said, "Oh, Daddy, don't do that. I don't need you to carry me anymore. I can run." It was my favorite moment at camp.

Even though we only have those kids for a week, we have had them for the week that is probably the most important week of their year. Somehow, you are connected. Even though it is a short time, I'm connected with them in a way that is much different from other adults that are in their lives. If things are good, they want you to know about it. If things aren't so good, they fall back on you a little bit. Some just move on

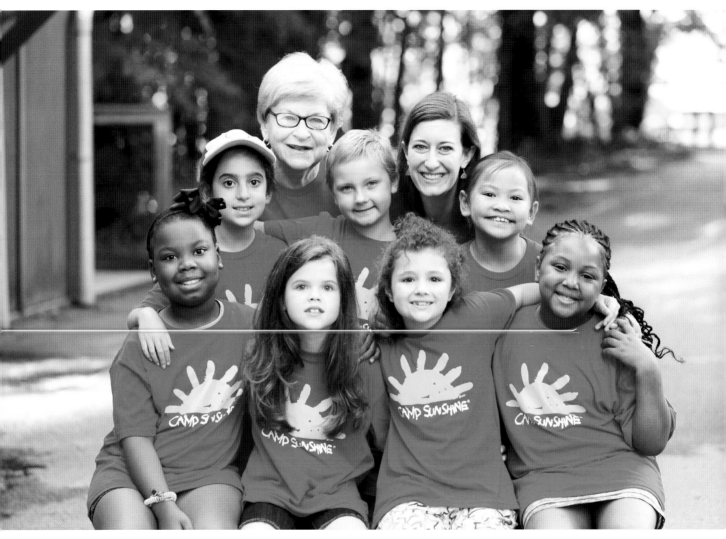

Jane (back left) with Stephanie, as cocounselors with their cabin

with their lives, and that is just perfect. For the people that need support and connectedness, I will always be available to them.

I still go to camp because it's the way I get recharged every year. If things are not right in the real world, for a week you turn off your phone, don't listen to anybody else's opinions about anything else. I am just there, in the moment, doing what people do for other people.

Camp is special—it is sort of like that little magical moment where you get to be the best you can be and hopefully help other people be their best too. When I raise money for Camp Sunshine, I say, "If you want to make the world better, make it better for these kids for a week." Because that is what happens here. The kids get it. They get camp's mission and what camp is about.

It has been a treat to have Stephanie as my cocounselor for the last five years. From the very first year, we have worked well together. Stephanie is mature for her age. She has been a camper. She is a physician. She gets this. By the third year of working together in our cabin, we reached that point where we almost didn't have to talk. We could see things out of the corner of our eyes, we could send messages without saying a word, and I loved that about her.

Stephanie is observant and kind and is supportive to the kids. She sees things that need to be done without anybody having to mention them. She keeps the kids safe and yet gives them lots of freedom. Stephanie is always willing to try to help. I just enjoy her as a person.

Stephanie has made me a better team player. I quit worrying about camp when Stephanie became my cocounselor. I know that I can count on her, and together, we can keep those kids safe, and we can make sure they have a good time and that they get to know each other.

It is that routine that you see in life that's good, with people that you know and trust, that makes our relationship special. It's that consistency, that stability that I love to see in Camp Sunshine.

7

They care because they've seen it

David Tardif (September 22, 1976–February 4, 1994; hometown: Lawrenceville, Georgia), as told by Marc Tardif, and Duncan and Kappi Dobie

MARC

I was exposed to Camp Sunshine because of my brother. Thinking back to the timing of David's cancer diagnosis, there were four of us growing up together. I have an older brother, Dominic. About a year later there is me. Three years after me, my little brother, David, comes. Then in three more years, I have a little sister. I had just left for college, so it's 1991.

We were all tennis players. We lived in a neighborhood where you could get to the tennis court by bike, so that is something that we did often. David was really good at it. I remember he hurt his leg that fall and thought it was a sprain. He was not sure what it was, but he just played through it. He did not complain much about those kinds of things in general. When I came home from college around Christmastime, his leg bothered him enough to have it looked at. When the doctors took X-rays, they found something in his leg, and they thought it was serious and had to be looked at further. From there, David saw an oncologist. Pretty quickly, he was diagnosed with osteosarcoma and started treatment. That was at the end of 1991. David would have just turned fifteen in September.

David's first camp program was the D.C. trip. He came back from that changed, and he had stories for days about all the things he had done in D.C. People were visiting him in the hospital and introducing him to the idea of going to camp long before he had gone on the D.C. trip, though. Steve Davol would stop by and visit in the hospital, and I would hear stories about Ron Williams and Steve, especially because they also had amputations and prosthetic legs. Their perspective was that if you are an athlete and you want to be able to do things, then a prosthetic is a much better way because knee rebuilds were not as strong or possible with below-the-knee amputations.

David's oncologist at the time was Dr. Vega. Dr. Vega told us that, in the same sitting when he described David's treatment, there was a camp for kids and teens with cancer, Camp Sunshine. I remember my mom—a nurse by training—had the mindset of fighting, that we were going to methodically get through this by doing the treatments. I don't think she was receptive right off the bat to David going off to camp, but pretty quickly, she came around on the idea. David went to Camp Sunshine in 1992.

David was older so it was different from having a young child in the hospital. My parents would visit David or stay with him during the day, but there was some independence also. My dad would stop by for an hour after work but then go back to the house. Being fifteen or sixteen, David did not feel like he needed someone sitting in his room or that he needed to have someone sitting side by side with him all the time. Even so, I felt a tug to home when I was at the University of Georgia. I was coming home from Athens on weekends quite a bit during David's illness and treatment.

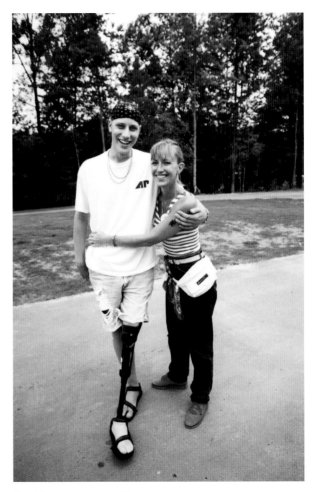

David at teen camp with counselor

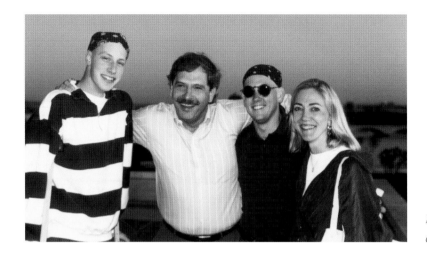

David (left), D.C. trip with Jay Beck,
counselor; Steve Davol, camper; and Sally

I remember every once in a while my friends from school and I would drive in from Athens and go out in Atlanta. We would stop by the hospital, hang out with David, and then go out in Atlanta and then head back to Athens. I checked in occasionally, but not all the time during my freshman year of college.

For David, the diagnosis of osteosarcoma meant treatment and the routine of staying off his leg or getting ready for chemotherapy. Even though David went to a big high school, there was no one who had had the same experience. After David came back from the Camp Sunshine teen trip to Washington, D.C., he had

other friendships. If you go to camp, everybody has the same experience.

People at camp get it, and it's easier to talk to them about it. Maybe it is just that you let your guard down a little bit more at camp, whereas you have been self-conscious at school about not having hair, about not being allowed to wear a hat, or wondering if you can wear a hat and get away with it. David did not have to worry about that kind of stuff at Camp Sunshine.

Camp is about sharing that common experience and a level of excitement about something. When Steve and Ron would visit or when David came back from D.C.

and had those exciting stories, there was something exciting happening, as opposed to just treatment.

While David was a camper, I got to pick him up and drop him off at camp. He would often say, "Come early, but we'll stay for a while before we drive back to the house. I want to introduce you to some people." A lot of them were other kids, and a lot of them were counselors also. I got to know several people. They were fun, exciting, and had good energy. After David passed away in February 1994, many of them came over to our house after the funeral. I remember Kappi Dobie and her husband, Duncan, taking a minute to say, "We think you should apply to be a counselor at Camp Sunshine." They were very supportive of my volunteering and encouraged me to do it, so I did, even though I felt nervous and uncomfortable going for the interview.

The summer after David passed away, my sister and I visited summer camp for a few hours one evening. We saw David's friends Karl and Steve, and everyone we knew there. I was comfortable there, and it felt like a great place to be. That is when I decided that it would be a good place to volunteer.

I first volunteered at Camp Sunshine the year after David passed away, in the summer of 1995. I have volunteered every year since, except for the summer my daughters were born because they were still in the hospital during the week of camp. After that, I went every year, and it has been twenty-three years now that I have been involved with camp.

My dad volunteered too. In the late 1990s or early 2000s, my parents moved to Connecticut. My dad came down for a few years and volunteered at the horse barn and was the activity staff for camper horseback riding. Then they left for Europe for several years, but when they moved back to Connecticut, my dad decided to go back to camp again and loved it. It was a family commitment.

My dad loves people in general. He loves to connect. At the barn, the kids that love it are a little bit different type of kid—the type that volunteers to wake up before breakfast and help out feeding the animals or brushing the animals. They are less likely to be the kids that want to hop up and down as much and more likely to want to be somewhere where they can take some time, cuddle by the fire, and just be with other people. I think my dad likes that part about being at camp. It was making connections with those quieter kids.

My dad still misses it. He still shares stories about the kids too. He helped certain kids get on the horses and watched to make sure somebody with a balance problem would be able to stay straight above the horse. He was able to get certain kids onto a horse when it seemed impossible. He had that patience and the knowledge to be able to do that. That was definitely a gift.

For me, it is the walks between the dining hall and the quiet times in the cabin or sitting on the porch in the evening that has made camp unique. Those are the opportunities *when the magic happens*, whether it is between campers or between counselor and camper. Those moments aren't scheduled. That's what camp is about.

Looking back at the twenty-something years as a volunteer counselor, it's funny because I have had almost the same role since I started. Scott and I have been cocounselors for several years, in the same cabin together with different ages of teenagers. I have always loved being in the cabin. You get more "camp" in those special quiet moments than you do in some of the other camp activities.

That first cabin we had from ages thirteen through eighteen was special. The kids were a lot of work, but they were great. That is what I liked about it: I stayed busy. We were constantly moving, taking care of things, thinking through challenges. Thirteen- and fourteen-year-olds are different from the older adolescents; they're a lot less independent, and they want to spend more time with their counselors, so you're more involved. That is what makes the great memories.

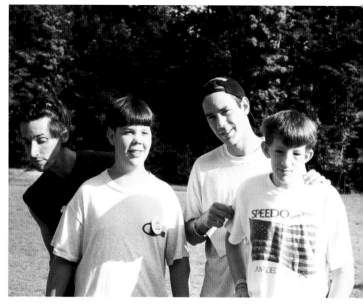

Marc (back right) with cocounselor Scott and campers

Will was part of that first cabin. He was a nice kid, well liked but not necessarily the most popular kid at camp. One year, he made it his goal to be the prom king, and he made it! I remember Will wore his crown all day, throughout the rest of the week, even on his last day. It meant that much to him.

Adam was another camper in our cabin. He was legally blind, and it took us a while to figure out exactly how much or how little he could see because he wanted to do so much. One day we were in the dining hall. We did not know everybody very well yet. Back then, the kids got up and served themselves, family style, from a platter. Adam volunteered to go get the platter. Once he had gotten up, it took us a few seconds to realize, *Is he going to be able to see his way back?* He made it. All of us counselors wanted to get up and hover to make sure he would be able to clear it all on his own. But we gave him space and encouragement, and he made it!

Sometimes the cabins reconsolidate when the campers are fifteen or sixteen years old. They break up or mix with other cabins when fewer kids come to camp or when the cabins are smaller. One year we had a reconsolidated cabin and a new sixteen-year-old camper who was not excited about being at camp. He came with a story about having to leave on Tuesday because there was an exam he had to take, so his parents were going to come pick him up. He was going to give camp a try, but no doubt on Tuesday, his parents were going to come pick him up.

That first evening is always a little bit hard for the new campers. They don't always want to be there, but they get over that quickly. This camper made a call home on the second day of camp and said, "I think I can leave on Wednesday and still be OK for my exam."

He stayed an extra day. Then it was another call to say, "I think I can be OK until Thursday if you come around dinnertime. I can still make it home for my exam then." Eventually, his parents did show up on Thursday, when the camp dance was scheduled. He made them sit on a bench during the entire dance because he did not want to leave until it was over. It is just funny to see how a new camper changes; once they are at camp and get into things a little bit, they fall into the camp rhythm, and it becomes really hard to leave.

I still see it with new kids all the time. We always say that by Wednesday, kids will hit their stride. Those first couple days are hard. This year, we were a little worried at the beginning of the week, about one of our campers falling into the swing of things. He was older. But by Tuesday or Wednesday, everything had fallen into place, and we had a rhythm. We were like, *Why do we even question the system? Why do we even have doubts on Monday or Tuesday?* It is hard to assimilate, but then, it just happens. You know it's going to happen. You just have to keep everybody rolling, and it always works out in the end.

To me, the connection to camp is having somewhere to go to remember David without necessarily talking to people about him. It is not a focus, but it is nice to know that many other people remember him or have good

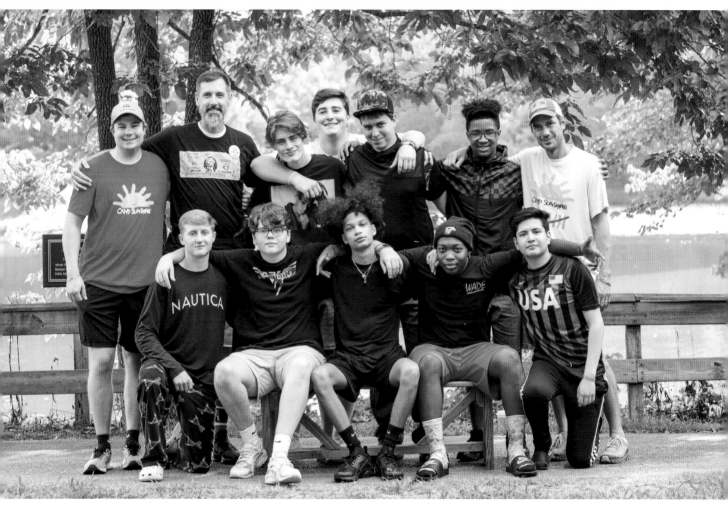

Marc (right) with Scott and their cabin

experiences from knowing him back when he was in the hospital or at camp. Every once in a while, I learn something about David from someone that I never would have guessed knew him. They will say, "Oh, I remember your brother." Sometimes it'll be decades later—ten, fifteen years later—and they will say, "Oh, I knew your brother from the hospital. I used to be in IT." For me, it is just nice to be around people that knew David and what brought me to camp.

Camp Sunshine is a community. The kids go home with relationships with other people who know what they are going through. It was a little bit of an epiphany the first year I saw David go to camp. I watched him leave and then return from camp super excited about how he was one of the special campers, one of the best new campers. His counselor had given a speech and had given him his award and went on about all the things David accomplished during the week and how special and different David was.

When you go as a counselor, you realize *oh my God, everybody goes home feeling that way*. It's built into the way camp operates, that being the most special child was not specific just to my brother. Had I never been a counselor, I do not think that would have ever clicked. David was the best camper. He was. But so was everybody else. They all feel that way.

Volunteers who have been going for so long are really a testimony to the organization; we are all committed to what camp is about. It is powerful.

David's friendship with Duncan and Kappi Dobie was special and is significant to our family. We share a lot of good memories of David, like the second year that David came to camp, when he essentially "broke himself out" of the hospital to come. He had some chest tubes draining from a lung surgery he had. The doctor said, "Absolutely not before Friday or Saturday will we release you." Somehow, we were able to get his chest tubes pulled early, which meant he had recovered a little bit quicker than expected, and he came home on Wednesday. Our mom let me drive him up to camp on that Wednesday or Thursday evening. I remember walking through the arts and crafts building with him when we arrived. Kappi was there. She looked up at him, and her face just went flush. She said, "What are you doing here!?" She was excited to see him but so surprised! It was so important to him to go to camp that he had to get up out of the hospital to get there, and he did. He stayed up late that night and told stories, and we came home, and he slept for a day and a half straight.

The summer of 1994, David went with Camp Sunshine to Colorado for an outdoor adventure program.

Duncan Dobie and another camper were on that trip; the three of them would wake up early and make breakfast before anybody else was up and would stuff pinecones under each other's sleeping bags. David had his leg amputation and started with his prosthetic but would not have been wearing it all the time, still using crutches. There were a lot of challenges to hiking and rock climbing on that trip, but David was able to do a lot of it. On the morning of the group's big peak ascent, the kids talked and decided where they were going to go and how they were going to do the hike. They planned their hike knowing that David, with his fairly recent amputation and prosthetic, would be challenged on rough ground, and they made it. I think that must have been empowering.

I recently had the opportunity to tell someone about camp. There was a young boy in golf camp with my daughters. He was too young to go to camp but had been diagnosed with cancer and finished treatment. I was talking to his mom and I had my camp T-shirt on. I didn't want to push it too hard, but I told her, "Camp's wonderful, and it is definitely something you should look into." People always have apprehension. I felt like this boy's mom was ready to move on. I said, "This is something you need to do for your child, even after he is through with his treatment. It's an opportunity for

him to connect with other people who understand. It fills some need that kids who are off treatment have."

If David were here today, I think he would say the same thing. He would say that Camp Sunshine is one of the most wonderful places on Earth. There is a video of Steve and David sitting on a log being interviewed for a news outlet, and David said camp is a place where he could feel comfortable with himself.

If you look around a cabin of campers, that's exactly what you see: kids at the same age from all over the state and very different backgrounds, and they fall together. In no time, they're getting along beautifully without any counselor involved. That almost happens on its own. It's amazing to see.

Several years ago, Herb and I had a cabin together. He told me that one of our boys had been avoiding his physical therapy for rehabbing a knee. I think nurses, doctors, and physical therapists had been encouraging him to do his physical therapy, and he wasn't doing it. The camper was sitting there telling the other boys in his cabin, "My doctor told me that if I had been doing my physical therapy, I'd probably be walking by now." These fourteen-year-olds got dead serious, and they responded, "Are you kidding me? You need to get on that!" They were the ones who laid down the law. "You need to get on your physical therapy. You need to be walking by the time you come to camp next year." By the end of the week, the camper was walking his wheelchair instead of sitting in it. It was funny. Because the kids care, even if they've just met. *They care because they've seen it.*

DUNCAN

During my family's experience with camp, we came to know David Tardif and a lot of different campers through the years and to know their stories intimately. We watched them grow up! The stories of Camp Sunshine, the relationships that are formed there, and the bonds, are incredible. The connection volunteers feel toward these campers, toward each other, is an incredible bonding experience, and it comes together like an endless circle.

My Camp Sunshine story began at Christmastime in 1974 with my wife, Kappi, and our daughter Katherine. Back then, there were no pediatric oncologists in Atlanta, not at Egleston or Emory or anywhere. Katherine was six years old and in the first grade when she became very sick in early December. She had a wonderful pediatrician who was in his eighties, Dr. Cathcart. He recommended having some blood tests done. After the testing, an adult doctor diagnosed Katherine with acute lymphocytic leukemia (ALL). I remember he was sitting there smoking a cigarette when he said, "Your daughter has leukemia." He told us there was nowhere in Georgia to take her. We started the search, and we decided on St. Jude's Hospital in Memphis, Tennessee. At that time, the diagnosis was bleak, almost a death sentence. Outcomes were nowhere near what they are today. I remember asking the doctor at St. Jude's, "Do you think you can get her in remission?" He answered, "Yes, for a while," but he did not paint a rosy picture.

Katherine's initial protocol was three and a half years of chemotherapy. She went into remission almost immediately. Then, in mid-1978, she relapsed several months after going off treatment. So it was back to St. Jude's for more treatment. It is incredible to think just how far treatment has come in the years since Katherine was diagnosed. Like most children today, she was treated on an outpatient basis. Bone marrow transplants weren't an option back then, so when Katherine relapsed at age nine, she basically had to go through the entire treatment protocol—chemotherapy for three more years—again. At the end of her second round of treatment her doctors told us, "We have some new drugs that are working wonders, and we'd like to give her one more round just to be sure. If there are any bad cells in her body, we want to get rid of them once and for all." So she lost her hair for the third time at age twelve. Katherine was finally released from treatment in 1985—eleven years after her initial diagnosis.

Katherine was one of the original Camp Sunshine campers in the summer of 1983. When we heard a new camp was starting—a camp for kids with cancer—we encouraged Katherine to go. She was still on treatment at that time. That was the beginning of our relationship with Camp Sunshine.

On the day camp started, we dropped Katherine off. I told Sally Hale and Dorothy Jordan that I was intrigued by the idea of a summer camp for kids with cancer. At that time, it was practically unheard of. I told them that I was a photographer. When I asked if I could come back and take pictures of the kids at camp, they agreed, and so I was there for three, four, five days taking pictures of these kids and the incredible camp experience. To be able to photograph these extraordinary kids in this very picturesque setting with the grounds and the lakes . . . it's just hard to relay what a privilege it was. I couldn't leave it. Nighttime would come, and I didn't want to leave. It was a magical week.

As magical as it was for me, it was even more so for Katherine. Kappi and I saw a transformation in her that all parents would want for their child, especially one who has been through as much as she had been through. I believe this transformation was much the same for all the campers. Through photography, I got to know several of the campers very well. These kids had the time of their lives! When that week came to an end, it was very emotional for everyone. Everybody was crying and hugging; nobody wanted to go home.

The second year of Camp Sunshine, 1984, I went for the whole week of camp to take pictures. I told Kappi, "You've just got to go too. This is an incredible place, and you have to go and be a part of it." It wasn't hard to convince her because of all the friends Katherine had made and the tremendous transformation camp had had on our daughter. From then on, our connection with Camp Sunshine as a family just grew and grew.

After several years we started doing a yearbook, taking pictures of every single camper who came to camp each year. The yearbook became a big project. Looking back, those early yearbooks were so primitive; that was back in the days when we had to convert color slides into black and white photos. But for me, it was just a wonderful opportunity to photograph these campers. Many of the kids started going to camp when they were seven years old, and they went back every year until they were eighteen years old. Some have gone on to become camp counselors themselves, so I got to see them grow into adulthood. Many beat cancer, were considered cured and cancer-free, and went on to live full lives. I've seen them go off to college, get jobs, and begin careers. I've seen some of them get married and have children of their own. Camp has given me the unique opportunity to know these extraordinary people.

Sometimes I can't believe that Camp Sunshine has been around for more than thirty-five years, but then again, maybe that's because camp has never been stagnant. Camp Sunshine leadership were always thinking, *What are we going to do next year to be different? How are we going to make this even better for these kids?* Camp was always expanding. Take the Washington, D.C., trip in 1986. The things we got to see and do in Washington were incredible! Special tours of the FBI, special tours of the White House that nobody else could do . . . behind the scenes stuff. When people realized these kids had cancer, they couldn't do enough for them. I believe I went on the D.C. trip for eighteen years. I joke with people that I've been in the White House more than some politicians!

Years ago, I wrote a story about David Tardif, but I never finished it. It was going to be in the form of a Christmas letter . . . you know, the letters that people put in their Christmas cards. It's a story about who David was as a young man.

I met David in 1991. He had osteosarcoma and had just had his leg amputated, but he was up and around and about like nothing had happened. At seventeen years of age, he was truly a brilliant young man. He was a straight A student who could talk about anything with anybody. He was very popular in high school, very likable, and an amazing young man. And he was fighting cancer, was on crutches, had had his leg amputated—and he was ready to go! Any kind of life adventure and he was ready to take it on.

Through camp, David became very close friends with Steve Davol (whose story is included in this book). Like David, Steve was battling osteosarcoma. Steve passed away in 1997, two years after David. Steve had taken David under his wing and had become his mentor. They were both amputees. During David's first year at camp, Steve took it upon himself to show David all the ropes.

I was very fortunate to know Steve and David and for them to be so close to my family. I was a chaperone on a Camp Sunshine outdoor adventure trip to Colorado with David only a few weeks after his amputation. It was a rugged trip for him. We camped out in the wilderness, cooked over the open fire, hiked, and went rock climbing. It was hard work. But I can tell you, I never laughed so hard in all my life. David and

Danny, another remarkable camper who was along on the trip, were full of pranks, full of life. They'd put rocks and pine straw in my sleeping bag. They were so funny; they kept everybody in stitches.

I have a picture on my dresser of David rappelling down a wall from that trip. There was a huge rock wall at Camp Hale, the former home of the army's famed Tenth Mountain Division during World War II (now a state park). The kids would go rappelling or rock climbing on this wall, ninety or one hundred feet of sheer rock. David was standing there asking, "Should I use my prosthesis or take it off and just use my one leg?" That one leg had become so strong. But David decided it would be best to rappel down with his prosthesis on, and he conquered that wall! It was such a great victory for him! It was one of the scores of magical moments I've experienced being a part of camp.

As I got to know David, I also got to meet his family, and at some point, I met his older brother Marc. Marc had heard a lot of stories about camp from his brother, and he would pick David up from camp and camp programs. After David died, Marc began volunteering. He became a fixture at camp; he was always there for summer camp, always ready to help out. Whereas David was very outgoing, Marc is on the quieter side. But he commands a lot of respect from the campers,

his fellow volunteers, everybody. He is not in the limelight, but he doesn't need to be. He is always there for Camp Sunshine, and his campers absolutely love him. Everything he does at camp, he does in memory of his younger brother. It is a wonderful way to honor David's memory.

Marc's years of volunteer service and his contributions to camp are a real testimony to David and to the ties that bind people who are touched by camp. Camp means so much to so many people. When David's cancer started coming back, it came back to his lungs. The week before camp started, David had to have an operation on his lungs, so we didn't expect him to be there. But knowing David, we should have expected differently. He was out of the hospital one day, having had major surgery on his lungs, and he showed up at camp! I was staying in a room in the infirmary, and Sally asked me if I would stay in that room with David. Of course, I would. David spent a day or two at camp just walking around, talking to his friends, and having a good time.

David passed away soon after this final trip to camp. At David's funeral, the Tardif family asked me to speak. It was a big honor for me. There were so many young people there. About half of them were David's friends from Brookwood High School in Gwinnett County and half were friends from Camp Sunshine. He was as popular at school as he had been at camp. Everyone knew his plight, everyone was in his corner, and everyone was absolutely torn up at the funeral.

At the funeral they said there were grief counselors on hand for anyone who might need those services. But Steve Davol said, "This is not good. David would not want all his friends being so sad. Let's get these people laughing; let's get these people talking about David and telling David stories." So that's what we did. Everybody spent an hour and a half telling funny stories about David's life. Steve had started something really big, and everyone left with smiles on their faces thinking about David.

Marc said his brother would describe Camp Sunshine as "one of the most wonderful places on Earth." Yet, it is also a camp for kids battling these incredibly difficult diseases. When we started going to camp all those years ago, we realized it was something we wanted for our daughter. Katherine had been through so much in her life, and we wanted to give her the chance to function well in society, to have friends, to have normal childhood experiences, and to have the experience of summer camp. Camp Sunshine gave her all that and so much more. Today, Katherine is doing great. She lives on St. Simon's Island, where she has her

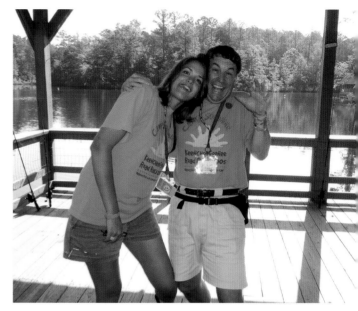

Duncan (right) with Kelly

own landscaping business. A lot of her clients live on Sea Island; they absolutely love her.

Camp changed my life, too, from the very first year I was there with my daughter. Camp Sunshine has made me the person I am today. The relationships I have formed and the people I have known, wonderful people like Steve and David and Marc, have influenced my life in countless ways.

Camp is so special and powerful. I often hear these kids say, "I have cancer; I get to go to Camp Sunshine!" They look forward to it every single year. Then when they are eighteen years old and have to graduate, moving on is devastating to them. Of course, many of them do come back and go through leader in training (LIT) and become counselors themselves.

So many children with cancer don't necessarily like who they are because they think they look different or ugly. They lose their hair; they've had amputations; they're using prosthetics. At camp, none of that matters at all. I remember years ago meeting a young girl named Jessica; she was twelve or thirteen at the time and had been diagnosed with leukemia. She was baldheaded that summer, and I would tell her, "Jessica, you are so beautiful without your hair!" And she was. Years later, I bumped into her and she told me, "I'll never forget what you told me. You said I was beautiful even without my hair." Those are the kinds of stories you hear from camp all the time. You just never know whom you are going to influence in your life.

Everybody at camp, people like Marc Tardif and all the volunteers, make these kids feel special. And when they leave camp, they know they are special in the eyes of so many people. And it's this specialness they carry with them every day. It is just amazing when you think

about the hundreds of children—no, the thousands of children and their families—who have been touched by this magical place.

KAPPI

Marc is a special person. I always look forward to seeing him. It's a connection that's important to me. He went through a lot as a young man, having lost his brother and seeing his parents go through the heartache of losing a child. Because of these experiences, you could see that Marc had an immediate empathy for the other campers and their families. Marc had an immediate understanding, a true recognition of what these kids and these families are going through. He brings his special memories of his brother, the experiences he had, and his own capacity for caring to Camp Sunshine.

At the end of 1974, our daughter Katherine was diagnosed. I remember we spent New Year's in the hospital. Katherine was six years old, and she just wasn't feeling well. She wouldn't recover from the cold we thought she had. This cold went on and on and on. We had been to the pediatrician so many times, and finally, they decided to draw blood. To hear the words, "Your child has cancer . . ." I can't begin to describe that experience. It was an unbelievable time in my life. But I knew, *you must go through it, you must*. So I got through it one day at a time. That is the only way I could get through it.

In between Katherine's hospital stays at St. Jude's, her drugs were sent to an adult oncologist in Atlanta, and that's where she would receive her medications. There wasn't any choice but to see an adult oncologist. And I can tell you that was challenging. They had no experience in finding little bitty veins or injecting needles into little bitty hands.

That all seems like a lifetime ago. But when your child is so sick and fighting leukemia, all you can focus on is their treatment, their care, their physical health, their survival. You cannot focus on the other parts of their childhood and what they might be missing. And that's where Camp Sunshine came into the picture.

Duncan and I were involved in the Leukemia Society, and Katherine's name was on the first list of children who might benefit from Dorothy Jordan's idea about a camp for kids with cancer. Dorothy called us about it. We were very interested. The idea was not brand new, but it was still pretty new at the time.

Camp Sunshine does a wonderful job with their outreach to families. But in those days, back in the beginning, it was different. There was no Camp Sunshine experience to draw upon. There was no past experience they could tell parents specifically about Camp Sunshine. I remember calling Dorothy back and asking her lots of questions. "Who was going to take care of these kids? How were they going to be taken care of?" Dorothy answered all of our questions. Our daughters, Katherine and Ashley, had been to a regular summer camp and had enjoyed the experience. So we decided to go for it. But we were also thinking, *Wow, what are we getting into?*

We knew camp was very special. That very first camp, Duncan wanted to go and take pictures all day long, and that's what he did. When he got back that night, as soon as he walked in the door, he said, "Kappi, you have got to see this. It is amazing. You have got to see it for yourself." The next year, I joined my husband as a volunteer, and in time, so did Katherine and Ashley. Our initial family commitment now spans more than thirty years.

I remember it rained a lot during that first year at camp! We were at Lake Burton then, and when it rained, the ground would get soaking wet. And because the ground would get soaking wet, it was not a smooth transition for these kids to get from one activity to another. *How were we going to move them around with some in wheelchairs, some with prosthetics?* Duncan had an suv, and I can remember him piling the kids into it and moving them around from one activity to another. I'm not sure how we did it, but we managed.

In those early days, I was a camp counselor for the little boys. When camp first started, they had difficulty finding male counselors. It seemed in those days that the men were all working and the concept of taking a week of vacation time to spend at a camp for kids who have cancer . . . it was just so new. So, for the first several years, I would go back as a counselor to the young boys.

As Camp Sunshine's reputation grew, there were eventually sufficient numbers of male counselors, and I took on other volunteer roles. I was a counselor for girls ages fifteen to eighteen, and then I headed up what was then called the counselors in training (cit) program, now known as lit. I have worked with the lit program for almost thirty years now, and it is through that role that I truly experienced the connections that camp creates. The lit program helps young people learn and experience as much as they can about Camp Sunshine and the campers, including spending time being a cocounselor. To see the ones who have been campers themselves grow into this role, to grow into becoming young adults, to grow in empathy and understanding are amazing things to see.

Things definitely have changed since those early days. But I can tell you what hasn't changed about camp. The commitment of the staff, for one thing. They are so devoted and loving to these kids. The counselors return year after year and give these children the chance to experience things—independence, self-worth, joy—they might not have experienced in a while because of their disease. So many of these kids don't have hair, have prosthetics, are very sick or are physically limited. Depending on how they have been treated at school or in their community, they can be made to feel they are different from other kids. I remember one time Katherine had a little friend who stopped coming over to our house when Katherine was first diagnosed. Her mother thought Katherine might be contagious! But I understand; that was a long time ago, and people didn't understand childhood cancer the way we do today. We know better than that now. There are so many reasons why these kids feel different in their day-to-day life. But for one week at Camp Sunshine they can be in an environment where they aren't different anymore. For one week, they are given the opportunity to feel normal and to experience joy and independence and self-esteem. Camp was and is all about making sure that children survive with these essentials intact.

I felt the significance of the camp community every time I went to family camp. At some point, the kids would go off to do their thing, and the parents would have their own session. Sometimes a doctor or maybe a nurse would come and talk to us. And I would be there as a kind of resource. There were so many parents who were still in shock that this was happening to their child, not even knowing which foot to put in front of the other. But having a parent there who truly knew what they were going through helped. It always made me feel good to be able to provide those parents not just with practical information but maybe something more . . . maybe empathy or hope . . . to see someone standing there who has gone through it.

As one of the lead counselors for teens, I worked with many of the girls for years in a row and got to know them well. When I started heading up the CIT program, it made sense for me to talk with Sally Hale and share with her an informed opinion about which campers I could see being a CIT. For me, the experience of seeing these young women—who I'd known as young campers—grown-up, mature, and becoming CITs was amazing. In many ways it was a miracle.

For my family, I believe camp has created empathy in all four of us. It has made us want to take our time to understand what someone else is going through. I

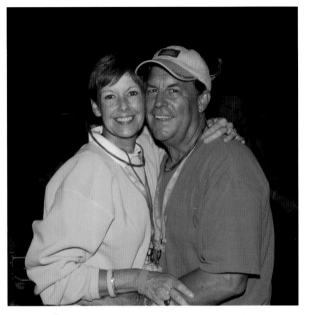

Kappi and Duncan

was brought up by very loving parents and taught to be kind and to help others in need. But being around these children and the entire camp family brings the idea of giving back to a whole new level. At camp, you are surrounded by other adults whose main purpose is to make sure these children have a safe and unforgettable experience at camp. All these volunteers want to do is give back.

Duncan was very close to Marc's younger brother, David. When David's cancer came back and he became very sick and was homebound, Duncan would go visit him once a week or more. I went with him toward the end. Duncan believed David was hanging on because he didn't think Steve was ready to lose him yet. David and Steve were so close. The day finally arrived when David told Steve, "I think you're ready, and I'm ready." He died the next day.

I remember seeing Marc and encouraging him to become involved in camp when he became ready to take that step. It is his personality to be caring. I told him he had a special knowledge, a unique and important perspective of what these families and children were going through, and it might be his gift to share it. What he experienced could give other families strength.

I have always been fond of Marc and his family. I felt a special empathy for his mother, Yvonne. As a mother, I could just feel the hurt in her. To see that pain and feel that pain in her . . . to see her in those last days of David's life . . . I just couldn't help but feel it myself.

I can't imagine never having experienced the love and joy between people that we find at Camp Sunshine.

It's the kind of love and joy that everyone needs in life. At camp, those children are trying to experience one more day in their lives . . . one more week in their lives . . . and they're trying to make it to the next summer so they can experience it all over again. They are going to grab it all, and that is a joyful, joyful thing to see.

Through camp we learn that we don't know what tomorrow will bring, and we can take these lessons learned at camp and apply them to the other parts of our lives. At Camp Sunshine, you can experience the joy these children have every day they are there. They have a zest for experiencing things that their diseases have taken away from them. They have questions like, "How long before I can be normal again? How long before I can do normal things?" Whether it's on the ropes course or in the arts and crafts room, they realize they can do "normal" things, things they weren't sure they would ever do again. They make full use of the limbs they do have and the strength they do have.

To know, even in some small way, that you can help a child do these things is life changing and life shaping. But you know what's even more amazing about camp? It's what these children do for us.

8

We are doing something right

Ansley Riedel (born October 22, 1987; hometown: Atlanta, Georgia)
and Nanci "Bubbles" Dubin

ANSLEY

We all say, "Camp, it's like magic." I was first diagnosed with acute myeloid leukemia (AML) when I was ten months old. I went through a lot of treatment and two relapses. I had my second bone marrow transplant at three and a half years old and have been healthy ever since. My baby brother was my donor for that second transplant, so that's a really special part of my story. My parents heard about Camp Sunshine through the hospital in Atlanta. I don't remember this, but we first started going to family camp when I was young, before my brother was born.

My parents have said that I was a very easy baby. I didn't fuss a lot and slept well. We were on vacation when my parents started realizing that I seemed a little bit more irritable than usual. I would fall asleep in their arms, but when they would lay me down, I would immediately wake up and start crying. I was more lethargic than normal and wasn't eating as well. It was that parent's instinct of *something isn't right*.

The doctor who examined me misdiagnosed me with pneumonia, but my parents knew, *no, that's not right*. They somehow stumbled across a pediatrician, who ended up treating me for the rest of my childhood. It was one of those chance moments where you stumble into a great patient-doctor relationship. This doctor didn't know what exactly was wrong, but he saw in my lab work that my white blood count was through the roof. He told my parents, "Take her to Egleston [Children's Hospital]. Go right now. Leave." I can imagine that was scary for my parents.

It's amazing that I have some memories of my treatment. Pictures help, but I remember spending a lot of time in my hospital room in Seattle (the site of my second bone marrow transplant). I remember the view I had of Mount Rainier. We called it my mountain. On clear days, which is sometimes a prayer in Seattle, we could see my mountain from the hospital room window. That was really cool to have. I remember funny things, like when we rented a cute house and my friend, a neighbor who was my age, would race pedal go-karts down the hill. We'd get to the bottom of the hill and my dad would push us back up and we'd go back down again. Probably not the best idea with my low blood counts and me being on treatment, but I had the best time doing that.

My younger brother, Joseph, and I are a little over three years apart in age. At four months old, he was my donor. He couldn't stay in the hospital, and he did not take a bottle, so it was hard for my mom to be in the hospital with me. She could not be away from him for too long because he had to nurse. But occasionally, we would bend the rules. We padded the bathtub so Joseph could sleep there, and my mom could spend the night. My grandmother Mimi spent a lot of time in the hospital with me, which was special too. My dad was back and forth working. It was a family affair.

The first memory I have of Camp Sunshine was during the summer when I was four. My parents took me for a visit. I knew that Camp Sunshine was a place where I would eventually go as a camper, and I was really excited about that. All I remember from that first year is a lot of wooden buildings and meeting Kati Tanner Gardner, who still goes to teen week as a counselor. I met her and some of the girls that were admitted to the hospital for treatment at the same time as I was. It was overwhelming. I was bombarded, overwhelmed by these campers who were so excited to see me and bring me back to their cabin. I was like, "I don't think so. No thanks. I'm good. I want to stay with my mom and dad."

I ended up visiting camp when I was five and six, too, so I have a couple of extra camp bracelets that I still wear and love. After those visits, I was totally ready to go to summer camp. I was excited. I didn't look back. I never felt homesick once, and it was perfect. I got over that feeling of being overwhelmed very quickly.

I have some funny memories of my first week at junior camp. My cabinmates were an entertaining group of girls. I remember some of them were still in treatment. We just had a great time. Thinking back now that I'm a counselor, I wonder, *What in the world were they thinking? How did we get away with this as seven- and eight-year-old campers?* Our dance theme was from the '80s, and I brought my Grandma Mimi's fluffy jacket

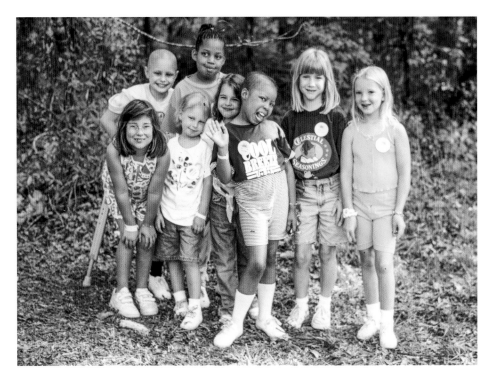

Ansley (far right)
with her cabin

and broad-brimmed hat with me to camp. There's a picture of us all lined up with attitude, our hands on our hips. I remember thinking, *I would never let my campers do this*. Well, now that I'm a cabin counselor with ten- to twelve-year-olds, maybe I would. Yeah, that first summer was so funny.

I had amazing counselors, Tricia and Verwray. They were influential as my first counselors and just hysterical. Verwray kept us laughing. Some of the campers were really messy, and some did not have any spatial awareness. She would make us giggle so hard talking about panties migrating across the floor. She would be like, "Whose are these? You better pick these up." I remember thinking, *I want to be a counselor. They are so cool. I want to do what they are doing.* Then as I got older, I realized, *I am going to graduate. I have to find a way to get back to camp. Duh, I will be a counselor. That is what I have to do.*

I remember loving the feeling of independence. We had choices for activities, and there were all these new things to try and do. To just have those little moments of freedom and independence to choose, to make decisions, was liberating. I remember in the evenings I would run ahead of the group and get back to the cabin before anyone else to get the first shower. I have no idea why that was so important to me. Maybe it is because I loved having the ability to do that, to do it on my own.

I loved having my bed neatly made, and I always brought my teddy bear, Hope Cuddly Bear, with me. One of my primary nurses gave him to me, and he always sat on my bed. My best friend, Kelly, would sleep in the bed next to me. Whichever of us got there first would save a bed for the other. Every night, Hope Cuddly Bear would fall off my bed, and every morning, Kelly would pick him up off the floor and hand him back to me.

I loved how we branched out to make new friends. Even though I had a core group of friends from my very first week at camp, each year I would have a new camper or two in my cabin. They would split some of the original cabins up a bit. I never knew the rhyme or reason, but it's special now to be a counselor with a lot of the newer campers and to see that progression of community and friendship.

I have thought about how there have been a lot of stages to camp and how it has changed yet somehow stayed the same over time. That love for camp and the connection that goes with it remains. When I was younger, camp was a lot about reconnecting with my friends once a summer, once a year, and getting to know them and the counselors. In some sense, it didn't feel like any time had gone by, even though, of course, a whole year had.

When I became a teenager, a new Camp Sunshine world of retreats opened. I could see my friends more than just once a year, and we would stay up, not all night but close enough, just talking and laughing and giggling. We would have a blast doing nothing. I loved having the chance to see them more than once a year. Even my friend Kelly, who moved away after the first summer of camp, would sometimes be able to make it to teen retreats from Colorado. Those retreats always went so quickly. Yet, at some points, time felt like it was standing still, like we could be there forever.

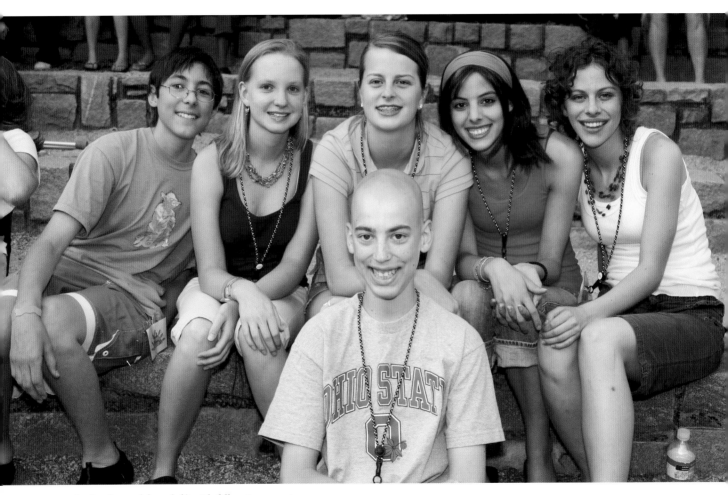

Ansley (second from left) with fellow teen campers

I never missed a summer. It was just not an option for me to miss camp! I started off with family camp and visiting camp then progressed through junior week all the way through teen week and into the leader in training role. That was a fun year for me.

The first summer I was a counselor in a cabin, I was twenty-two. I had wanted to be a cabin counselor. I wanted to have that bond with the campers and have that close-knit community that I had experienced with my counselors. Growing up, I loved the consistency of having the same counselors. I'm thirty now, and that's been important to me as a counselor, too, because I had such wonderful role models and loved seeing them every year. I enjoyed seeing them just as much as seeing my friends.

It is just so hard to put into words the importance of Camp Sunshine. My friends who have known me the longest, through elementary and junior high and high school, know how important camp is to me. I think sometimes, if you can connect with someone else who has had a similar camp experience, they can understand that drive and that connection that you experience at Camp Sunshine.

For others, it is so hard to explain what role the Camp Sunshine community has played in my life. It has been such a routine in my life for so long. I cannot

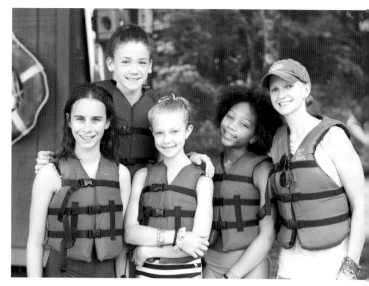

Ansley (right) as counselor with campers

imagine being anywhere else for a week in the summer or not volunteering at family camps and seeing Camp Sunshiners around town. It is not like I see people from camp that often. Although my closest friends and I see each other only once a year in the summer, we just have this instant reconnection.

My friends and I try to catch up and talk about our lives and our jobs and what we are doing, but there is a feeling of ease and comfort that we don't have to talk about the outside world. We put away all of our differences and beliefs and cell phones. It is so freeing to all be together and to have this same mission, to make this the best week for the campers. We remind ourselves that it is not our journey but the campers'. Camp Sunshine is all for the campers, and to have that shared goal of helping them is such a great feeling.

Bubbles has been an amazing friend to me and the most consistent connection I have had outside of camp. She always treated me like we were on the same level, like I was not a kid. We emailed a lot when I was growing up. She just gave me a book of all the emails I had sent her. I just rambled in all of those emails! I was all over the place, and I would tell her everything about school and my home life.

It got harder and harder to not be able to see my camp friends throughout the year. So many of them lived outside of Atlanta or outside of the state, and it was nice to have Bubbles close by. She was always that person right down the street from me. We would meet for dinner, she would pick me up, she would come to birthday dinners. She was always my camp connection.

We still got together when I would come home from college. She would take me to different restaurants in Atlanta. I tried sushi for the first time with her. Everywhere we went, she knew the owners, and we had special treatment. It was such a fun relationship to have. It was always hard to explain to my friends who she was because she is so much older than I am, although I didn't see her that way. I just saw her as this wonderful friend and woman to whom I looked up.

I have been a nurse at Children's Healthcare of Atlanta at Egleston for five years now. I work on the transplant step-down unit for solid organ transplants. I love it. I knew that I wanted to be a nurse because I have a lot of good memories of the nurses from when I was in the hospital. At the same time, I was fascinated by psychology and wanted to have a standard college experience. So, I ended up at Emory Nursing School as a second-degree student, after finishing my undergraduate degree at Sewanee. It took me seven years to finish my degrees. At times I thought, *I am so done, I am so tired of this, I could have just gone to nursing school. Why didn't I do that?* But my whole drive to be a nurse was from my experience as a patient. That bedside nursing role really touched me and inspired me, and it kept me motivated throughout my secondary education years.

Camp has been a part of my life for so long, and I have developed friendships with people from all over. I meet a lot of kids at family camp who are just starting their camp journey. I tell them about the friends I have met and the cabinmates that I have had and have kept in touch with since our first summer when I was seven, that we are now cocounselors together and have stayed friends all this time. I think that is helpful for the parents to hear, too, because we have a lot of timid parents who are thinking, *I am not going to make my kid go if they don't want to go.* I want to say, *Come on, push them a little bit harder. You will be surprised.*

I tell patients about the amazing friendships and connections they will make at camp. I tell them, "You don't have to say anything about your diagnosis, about your treatment, if you don't want to. It doesn't matter. We share a common understanding of why we are all here." In some shape or form, cancer has affected all of us.

In our cabin, campers go around the room saying, "I had this disease and I am two years off treatment," or, "I am still on treatment and I just relapsed." Some new campers who are actively on treatment, who were bald, would come to camp and wouldn't want to take their wigs off, but by the end of the week, they were like, *what wig?* It has always been a really, really, really great thing to see them get comfortable.

When I tell people about my cancer history for the first time, that I am a survivor, they are amazed and they want to know more, but I can tell that they don't have any idea of what that was like. I get a lot of sympathy. I do not need that. I don't appreciate it, but I let it roll because I know that that is the only way people know how to respond.

Sometimes I get the weirdest comments like, "Are you good now? Are you healthy now?" I think, "What do you think? Do you think I look healthy? Do you think I'm still sick? I'm twenty-seven years off treatment. Yes, I'm doing fine." With all the people I have met through camp, they just *know* what it is like. I don't have to go into it. We all know what we are dealing with, and we don't have to harbor it, work on it, or explain it. We just have that understanding. That is what makes Camp Sunshine so special. It is that common understanding, that unspoken bond that we have.

I had this marvelous, rewarding experience this summer. I was walking to one of the activities with two campers, one who was new and another who had missed camp last summer. Out of the blue, the new camper said, "I feel like I have been here for years." I wanted to shout and scream and cry happy tears because it was just such a great thing to hear her say. The other camper said, "Yeah, me too." It was so amazing. I downplayed it. I commented something like, "I am so glad you feel that way. That is a good thing for me to hear," or, "That is a good thing for you to say. I am so glad you are having a good time." The new camper replied, "Yeah, it means I fit in." I thought, *Oh, I am doing something right. We are doing something right.* I was so happy to hear that. It is so special. I love it.

BUBBLES

I have known Ansley since she was a toddler. I remember her when she was just a little girl—a cancer patient walking through the hospital in diapers! Years later, the first time I saw her at summer camp, it was such a joy to see her there as a first-time camper!

I remember Ansley always being there and being part of my life. I always wanted to be there for her too. She was often one of my campers at teen retreat, a weekend program during the year to help keep the kids "connected."

Ansley is surrounded by a loving family. Family is a huge part of her life. But she has always made room for others in her life, and I am thrilled to be a part of that. To this day, we stay in touch. We have an unbreakable thread between us, and whenever we talk or text or see each other, we pick up wherever we happened to have left off. I went to several of her birthday parties, her Sweet Sixteen, and her graduation party. We wrote

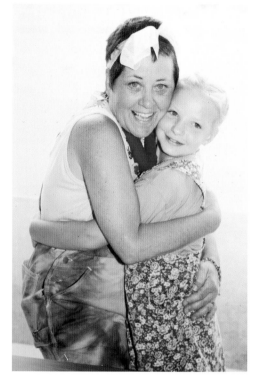

Ansley with Bubbles

letters when she was off at school. I cannot imagine my life without her or Camp Sunshine.

Because of camp, I am privileged to be a part of the lives of these wonderful people. I am a perpetual grandmother and, amazingly, a fairy godmother to many children of the campers, now grown, who I met at camp. I have been the flower girl at two campers' weddings. To me, this speaks to the continuous circle of love and dedication you find at camp. It never stops.

When you arrive at camp, it is like a family reunion. You are seeing family members who maybe you haven't seen in a year. But it doesn't matter. You just hug everybody, especially if you're me. You just give everyone a hug, and let the week begin!

In the early days of camp, we didn't have a specific detailed plan. But all of us knew we had this incredible desire to help these children, to give them a true camp experience and to give them a week to just be a kid again. I believe we have done this from the beginning. We pack more into a week of Camp Sunshine than other camps do in two and a half or even three weeks. I bless Dorothy for even having thought of this idea—this improbable idea—a camp for kids with cancer.

Camp is simply amazing. From the very beginning and still today, I would say that all of us volunteers simply drop our egos at the front gate, and then we have a love fest for a week. The size and intimacy of camp have changed. Camp used to be so much smaller where everybody got to know everybody. We were very close. Now with over 240 campers in one week alone, I can't get to know every single camper the way I used to. So, yes, you lose some of the closeness, but the upside is the number of children who can be served by Camp Sunshine nowadays.

Another thing about camp that doesn't change is the dedication of the volunteers. Camp has a very high return rate for volunteers. I have truly made some of the dearest friends I have ever had through camp. Love rules at Camp Sunshine. Camp itself has grown, but the love endures. It is one thing that never changes.

The day the Camp Sunshine House opened was an open house event. Sally Hale was welcoming everybody in. She said, *Welcome to your home*, and that is exactly what it felt like to everybody there. It felt like home and continues to feel that way.

Camp Sunshine helps instill a can-do spirit in children. I've seen children who are missing a limb climb to the top of the climbing wall; a blind teenager walk a tight rope; and kids who you think are too sick to participate in camp join in all the activities and love every minute of it. They have an indomitable spirit.

I'm an adult cancer survivor. If anything, that has strengthened my camp commitment. In a way, it was like *welcome to the club*. Not that it's a club you want to belong to. One thing I have learned through camp is you have to deal with whatever life hands you. You

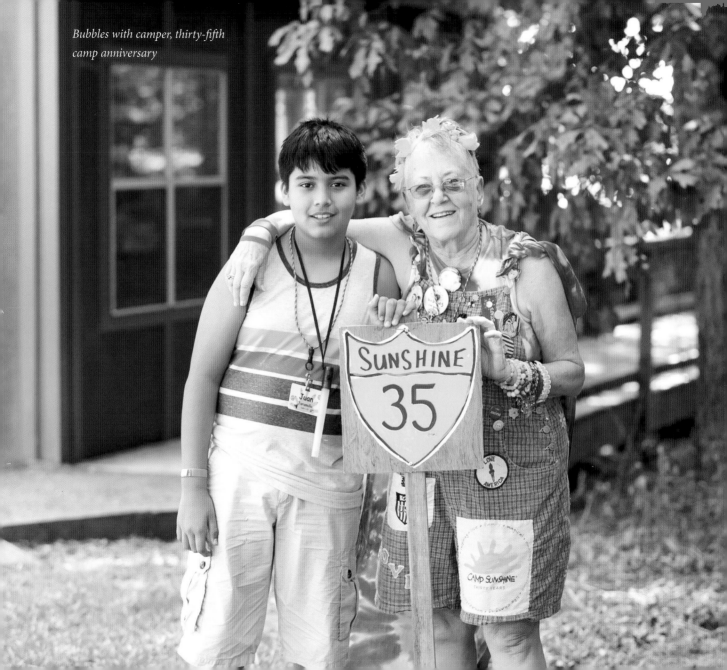

have to learn to go with the flow. I am fortunate to be surrounded by love on all sides, and I thank my lucky stars every day for all that love.

Camp gives children the right to be happy, to go on with their lives, to step away from cancer at least for a while, and to experience normal childhood things. They learn that life is more, much more, than cancer.

Away from camp, these kids and their parents and families are dealing day-to-day with the overwhelming concerns of cancer treatment, medical appointments, uncertainties, and such. These children need time away from all that. They need Camp Sunshine, and it has been my enormous privilege to be a part of that!

9 I am safe with them

Carrie Turner (born October 25, 1995; hometown: Columbus, Georgia) and Dawn Stys

CARRIE

I think it was November 15, 2011. The date 11/15/11 was my D-Day.

I fell asleep in math class the Friday before, and my teacher called my mom. It's a very small school so she had my mom's number. She said, "Something is wrong with Carrie. She's falling asleep in class. She has never done this before. She is not the kind of girl to do this."

I'm normally a very energetic person. I'm always going one hundred miles an hour, but I was so tired. It was a bone-deep hurt when I walked, I had super weird bruises on my legs, and I just wasn't acting like myself. My grandfather has a platelet disorder, so my parents said, "Well, let's go to the doctor to see what is going on. Maybe there is something going on here."

The doctor ran some tests, called back about two hours after I had left the hospital, and said, "Come on back. We're going to admit you directly to the oncology floor. Your blood count is bad." I had a platelet count of ten thousand and a hemoglobin of nine, which put me at extreme risk of internal bleeding. The doctor said, "Get to the hospital now." From there, it all happened super fast. The doctors started talking treatment and six months and cure, and I was thinking, *What are these words?* Finally, the doctor told me, "You have leukemia. I don't know what type, and I don't treat children, so I'm sending you to Atlanta." So off to Atlanta I went.

Looking back, it is hard to remember anything that was going on at that time, but I remember I was shocked. I knew what leukemia was, and I knew what it did. About two months before I was diagnosed, a boy in my older brother's class had been diagnosed with leukemia. But he was nineteen and nearly an adult, so it felt different for me. The weirdest things went through my head. I was thinking, *Wait, I have a math test this week. I can't miss my math test!* Then I realized, *Oh crap! My hair is going to fall out! Oh, this is bad.*

Once they looked at my counts, the doctors told me, "It is super aggressive. If we don't get you chemo within the next week, we don't know if you will make it to next year." I had just started tenth grade and gotten my license the week before, and it was very weird thinking, *Here I am at sixteen years old. I am supposed to be in my prime with lots of freedom. Now, I literally may not make it to seventeen.* It was a very surreal and out-of-body experience.

When I got to the children's hospital in Atlanta, I was told that I needed to "start treatment now!" They said, "We're going to schedule surgery to place your port. We're going to do a spinal tap to give you a bone marrow aspiration. We're going to give you your first dose of chemo. We're going to see exactly what we're dealing with." All we knew at that point was that I had leukemia. The next day, after the bone marrow came back, the doctors told my family that I had ALL T-cell (acute lymphoblastic leukemia T-cell), which we found out is rare for teenagers.

That time, I was in the hospital for just a week. I went in on Monday, was transferred to Children's Healthcare of Atlanta on Tuesday morning, and was released on Sunday morning. I came out of that stay with my first dose of chemo, which they injected in my spine while I was in surgery to place the port (port-a-cath). After that, my treatment lasted three years.

The doctors at my local hospital had already said they weren't comfortable treating a child. I thought, *Well, if you're not comfortable treating me, I'm not comfortable having you treat me. I'll stay where the experts are.* So my parents brought me back and forth to treatment, driving me three hours once a week from southwest Georgia to Atlanta. They worked it out where my dad went to all my treatments the first month. Then every time I started a new road map or had an important treatment, he would come. He came to my last treatment, which decided if I would go on maintenance therapy or not. Other than that, he stayed home to take care of my two brothers and keep food on the table for us. My mom tried to work, but she was trying to take care of me at the same time so that was just too hard.

Before my diagnosis, life was great. I was super involved in school. I was a hurdler for the track team and had been a dancer since age five. I was a cheerleader and cheer captain. Cheer is my passion, and my life was wrapped up in it most of the time. Those activities are what kept pushing me throughout my treatment. I couldn't hurdle anymore, but I finally convinced my parents to let me cheer again. The start of cheer season marked the start of maintenance, so I knew, *if I can get to cheer season, then I'll be good.* Cheer was my saving grace, other than camp.

I first heard of Camp Sunshine during my very first week of treatment. A woman from camp came into my hospital room after I had had surgery. She was wearing a red T-shirt with this big Camp Sunshine logo on it. She asked me, "Do you go to summer camp?" I had gone to some kind of camp— Girl Scouts, 4-H—every year, so I responded, "I love summer camp!" Then she asked, "Do you want to go to cancer camp?" I was like, "What is cancer camp?" I was thinking, *This is super weird. You're going to send a bunch of kids who are bald and on chemo into the outdoors? I mean, this does not seem safe.* The thought of it was strange to me.

The woman left me with that year's yearbook and a list of Camp Sunshine programs. She told me, "We're actually having a teen retreat this weekend, but you're not going to be able to go to that. Here's the stuff. Call us if you have any questions. Your nurses know all about it, so just ask them and go from there."

That was in November. I kept that yearbook and all the paperwork, and I ended up attending my first camp that next June. I didn't want to go, though. I got forced to go. My doctor wanted me to stop chemo for a week so I could go to camp. I thought, *No way.* In my mind, that one week was going to make a huge difference. I said, "I want to go to camp. I really do, but I don't want to jeopardize my health and not finish treatment on time." My doctor said, "You need this. I've seen it too much. Kids need camp." I replied, "But I need treatment, that's what I need!" He told me, "Well, I'm in charge here. I say you're not getting your chemo the week of camp. I won't order it. And if you show up, you're not going to be on the schedule for clinic." He said, "If you don't show up to camp, I'm coming to south Georgia and I'm going to drag you there myself." So I went to camp. My mom likes to remind me all the time now that "you didn't want to go to camp, but you love it, and you keep going back."

My first camp was in 2012. My parents drove me. They were usually comfortable sending me to camp, but this time they were thinking, *My daughter's still in active chemo. She's bald. We don't know if we're OK with this.* My primary nurse, Molly, was there when I arrived. She was super excited for me to be there, which eased my parents' minds a little bit.

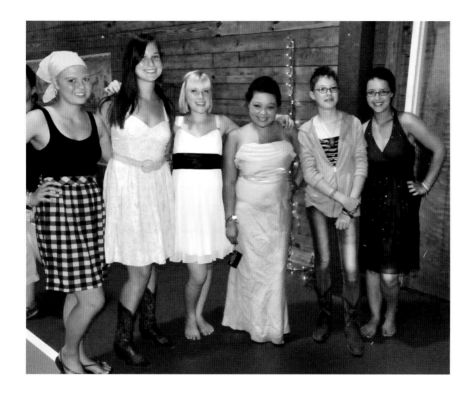

Carrie (far left) with fellow teen campers

Camp was loud. Music was blaring. Everyone was running around and hugging each other, screaming. I wondered, *Did these relationships happen in one week? There's a lot going on right here. There's so much to do. I'm going to be exhausted.* I was, and it was great. But at first, I was thinking, *This doesn't make sense to me.*

The campers were still bald. I could not wrap my brain around what camp was at that time.

My relationship with camp has gotten better and better every year. That first year, I was in a cabin of new campers. There was no veteran in our group, so we figured out camp together. We told ourselves, "Next

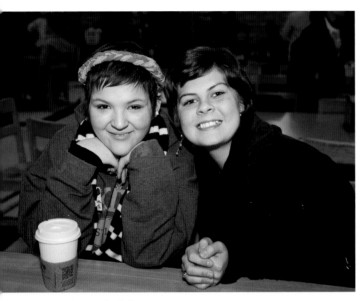

Carrie (right) at teen retreat

friends, and we were the ones saying, "Let's go and help the new campers that are coming in."

One of my best camp memories is from my senior year, when the new ropes course had just opened. My cabinmates had all agreed to go, and we got special permission to be on the course together, just us. We were shouting, "We love this! It is awesome!" We were on the very top rung when it started to lightning. The Camp Twin Lakes staff yelled up, "We can't let you finish with the lightning going on. We have to get you all down!" But the only way down was to finish. The staffers said, "All right, we are just going to have to break boundaries. You're going to have to rappel down from the top." They taught us how to rappel down under cover in time to get away from the lightning. It was intense, but we got it done. And it was very, very exciting.

Cabin chats at camp were always my favorite. Those were the moments when we got closest to each other. In just one week of the year, I got closer to my cabinmates than I did with the kids at school that I have been with since kindergarten. I talked to my friends from camp more than I talked to my friends from high school. The intensity with which we developed a bond was insane to me.

The whole point is that something negative like cancer can bring people together. I look at my friends

year when we come back, we will know a little bit more about what is going on and what we want to do." When camp came around the next year, we knew all the songs and the dances. You could tell we were no longer the weird first-year campers that everyone was trying to include. We had merged into the group. We were confident, "We know this, and we've got this." By the next year, when I was a senior, I had been on the D.C. trip, the teen retreats, and the lock-ins. I had awesome from camp and I know, *If I had met these people in college, I probably wouldn't have talked to them. They just don't fit the type of people I thought I'd be friends with.* Camp forces us to put aside our differences. Once you get talking to people, you realize, *There's a lot we have in common, even though it doesn't look like it.* I'm loud and flamboyant, but one of my good friends Harleigh is an extra step ahead of me. I probably would not have talked to her if I had met her outside of camp, but because of camp, our friendship works. It made it safe.

For me, the connectedness of camp extends past the campus. If I were out at Walmart and saw my nurses from the adult hospital where I was treated, I wouldn't run up and start chitchatting with them, as great as they were. If I see nurses from camp, though, I'm going to go up to them, and we are going to talk. Camp makes relationships take on a different meaning. The nurses aren't just my medical providers, and I am not just their patient. We are individuals on a different side of the same story, a different side of the same fight. We are all against cancer. The patients are against it because we are in it and it sucks. The nurses are in it because something in them has guided them to say, "I want to help these kids and I want to fight against cancer."

Pediatric oncology is not something that people like to talk about. It is very sad to people when they look at us, but being at Camp Sunshine, we know cancer is not the worst thing that could happen to us. We are thinking, *It could be worse!* We are just enjoying what we have. That first year of camp was very important to me, and I didn't realize how important until afterward. I had sunk into a hermit state; I was like a hermit crab. I didn't like going out because I was bald. I would say, "I am putting my bandana on and going to the grocery store, but that is it. I don't want to go anywhere else." I had just one friend that I was talking to; I wouldn't talk to anybody else because I felt like, *You are all being nice just to be nice at this point. You won't argue with me like we used to. Now you'll only agree with me. You are just doing that because I have cancer. You don't want to talk to me as your friend, but you want to talk to me because you are afraid I'm going to die in the next year.* I was a very social person, but I had sunk into this mode of, *I don't want to talk to anybody.* My phone stayed in my room all day. I didn't text; I didn't call. This was not like me. Camp brought me out of that depression. It gave me a reason to be OK with being the "cancer girl." Camp made me OK with the whole idea of having cancer.

Ever since then, I have looked forward to Camp Sunshine because camp is what gets me through to the next year. During nursing school, I wasn't able to go to camp because I was taking classes. I had to

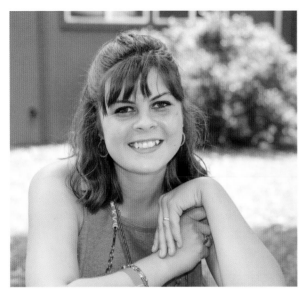

Carrie at teen camp

get through nursing school to go back to camp, to be able to transition from camper to counselor. I would pull up my pictures from camp. I wore my friendship bracelets to remind myself, *I have to get back to Camp Sunshine.* I had to get through whatever stage of life I was in to get back.

Camp is what keeps me going now even as a nurse. It drives me at work and at home. My boyfriend knows; I told him when we first started dating, "Camp Sunshine is a part of me, and it will always be a part of me. One week out of the year, I am going to camp. You have to take us both—Camp Sunshine and me. You can go with me or not, but I am going. You can't stop me." My parents know too. I work family vacations around camp events. I work my schedule around camp events. I already told my manager, "This is the week that I am going to request off next year." Everyone makes arrangements so I can go to camp because it saved me from being a super depressed loner when I was in chemo.

Growing up, I didn't want anything to do with the medical field. Cancer is the one thing that finally convinced me to be a nurse. Nursing is the only thing that sets my soul on fire, that keeps me going. So, I was super excited to become a nurse. About two or three weeks after graduating with my bachelor's in nursing, I decided I did *not* want to be stressing about NCLEX, the licensing exam for registered nurses, while I was at camp. I was like, *Camp is for camp, not for NCLEX.* So, I took the exam as soon as I could and found out on June 1 that I had passed and was officially a registered nurse. Then I went to camp and just enjoyed it.

After camp that summer, I started working in an adult emergency room. I realized quickly: *This is not why I got into nursing. I got into nursing to be in pediatric oncology. I have got to figure this out, or else I am going to quit nursing.* Now I work in a children's ER in Columbus. My goal is to eventually work in the Aflac Cancer and Blood Disorders Program at Children's Healthcare of Atlanta. I would love, love, love to be an Aflac Cancer Center nurse because Aflac is where I was treated. Aflac is what got me here. Aflac is the reason I went to nursing school and went through this mess. I have got to give back.

Some of the people who influenced me the most are my nurses Dawn and Molly. They encouraged me to go to camp, to become a counselor, and to be a nurse. Dawn was my primary nurse for my inpatient stays since my very first week of treatment. One night, she stayed *two hours* after her shift had ended to talk with me and explain to me and my parents what everything was. "This is what this count is. This is what it means." She impacted my treatment so much. Every time I was at the hospital, she would tell me what was going on at camp. She would always wear the camp shirt. She kept Camp Sunshine in my mind every time I was inpatient.

Molly did the same when I was outpatient. I saw Molly pretty much every week. She seemed to wear a Camp Sunshine shirt every time I was around her. After my doctor told me he was going to drag me to camp if I didn't go on my own, Molly said, "If he doesn't, I will!"

Before I left for camp the first year, Molly and Dawn both told my parents, "I will be there. I've got her." Even though they weren't my cabin counselors and neither of them were there as nurses, they were still "my nurses." They knew that their words helped my parents, and that helped ease me a little bit because I knew, *I am safe with them.* I trusted them to give me chemo, and I knew I could trust them to keep me safe at camp.

I don't want to say camp is everything because that is a little crazy, but Camp Sunshine is the most influential force in my life. Every year, I look forward to camp, and every week holds a little different bit of special magic. It keeps me going, it keeps me sane. I put my phone in my cabinet in the cabin, and it stays there. I come out to the fishing docks and sit in the rocking chairs and watch everyone and I think, *Yeah! I can go back to work next week and just be back to my normal self.* It helps me remember who I am and where I stand with everything.

If I didn't have camp, I would lose a huge part of who I am. I think about it sometimes, and it is almost sad, bittersweet. If there's ever a cure for cancer or we develop an immunization and get rid of cancer, that would be awesome. But then camp goes away, and I don't know if I am ready for that. I think, *I want cancer gone, but I don't want camp gone.* As long as cancer is here, camp is going to be here.

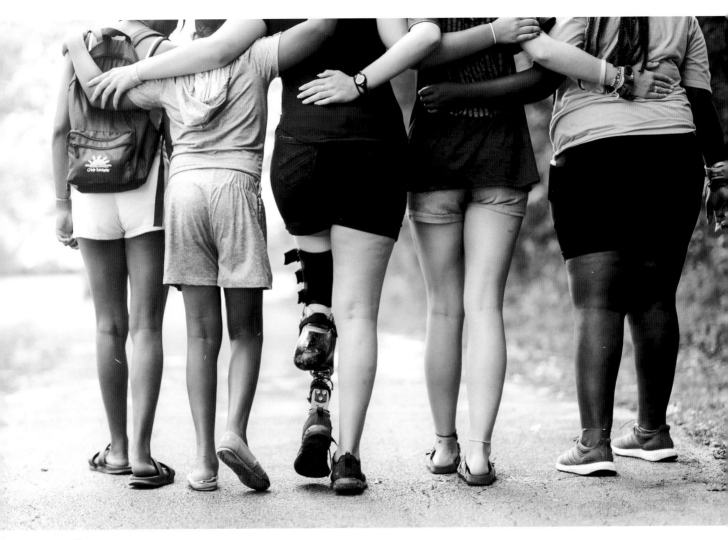

Teen campers

I think there's always a positive in every bad situation; every gray cloud has a silver lining. Camp Sunshine is that silver lining of cancer. Camp takes something negative and makes it positive. I look out from the dock at camp and see these kids on paddle boards who have had rotationplasty (a surgical procedure to remove a malignant leg bone tumor resulting in the appearance of a short leg with a backward foot). From the outside, everyone seeing these kids would be like, "Oh, man, how sad!" But at camp, these kids are running around with prosthetics on. It's something you have to see because it's indescribable.

I get asked all the time, "What do you do at Camp Sunshine?" I always say, "The same thing you do at a normal camp." This year, I had a new camper in my cabin. She did not want to get out of the car. She was tired, scared, and didn't want to go. I finally got her to stay for one night. I told her, "If you are going to be here, you are going to *be* here. We are going to live in the moment. We are going to be doing what people think is impossible for a cancer kid to do. You are a kid. You are taking back your life this week. Get ready!"

DAWN

This is my twenty-third anniversary at Children's Healthcare of Atlanta (CHOA). I started right out of school at the Aflac Cancer Center. I knew I wanted to do pediatrics. I was not sure beyond that as to which specialty, and I had a friend who worked on the oncology floor. We were in nursing school together, and she worked there as a tech. She was able to get me an interview. Long story short, I got a job. I remembered thinking, *Oncology, I don't know about this.* But it quickly grabbed my heart and was the start of my nursing career. That was in September 1995.

By June the next year, I had heard so much about Camp Sunshine that, of course, I had to go. My first summer at camp was in June 1996. I quickly learned that I couldn't do one without the other—just for the balance it gives me for the work I do in the hospital and seeing what the kids go through. Then to have that 180-degree difference at camp where they are normal kids getting to do normal things, having fun, and hanging with their friends. Just that magic that you don't see in the hospital! They sometimes can be completely different personality wise from one setting to the other. I love to see that because you just don't get to see their "light" in the hospital, but you do at camp.

I have never looked back or thought about doing anything else in my career. Every time a thought of a job change even flashes through my mind, I think this is what I love. This is a calling of sorts. People call it that, and I guess that is what it is. I just cannot see doing anything else. I feel the same about Camp Sunshine. I have had to take a year or two off over the years, and I just missed it. Those years felt very unbalanced for me. I quickly knew I needed to get back to camp.

There was some nervousness for me that first year, no hesitation, just a little nervousness, just not knowing what to expect, but total excitement from hearing all the nurses at CHOA talk about it. I went to camp as a kid off and on, but I knew this camp was totally different and knew the experience was going to be totally different. I was an activities counselor that very first year so that helped me get my toes wet and be a little bit on the outside of the boundaries of it and be able to take it all in. Yet, I still got to see all the kids that joined in those activities that I helped with. I was an activities counselor for three or four years before I became a cabin counselor. I filled the role of a cabin counselor for a number of summers before I became a unit head (head counselor).

Camp Sunshine wasn't what I expected it to be, in the best way possible. I expected camp to be fun.

I expected that there would be a lot of activities and things for the kids to do. But that intangible peace, that magic in a bottle, I never expected that! How the kids connect, how there's no bullying, and how they just love each other. It's crazy. To have that many years, and that many kids together, and it not to be about who is pretty, who is this, or who has these clothes on, that sort of thing like in a normal high school setting. You just don't have that. That I didn't expect at all. Things that I didn't expect were such a surprise, but a good surprise and what kept me going back.

When I think about camp my first year as a counselor compared to now, it was a lot smaller in scale. I remember our camp picture. We were able to take a picture of everyone all together in one shot! We took those pictures throughout the years of the entire camp, but there is no way we could do that now! Even though Camp Sunshine has gotten bigger, the essence of camp hasn't changed.

I remember that very first year learning the song "Love Is" and everybody singing the songs, and everybody knew the motions. I remember that distinctively and thinking, *What is this? I need to learn this!* I also remember looking around and just thinking, *Wow, look at all these kids. They already know this, and they are loving it.*

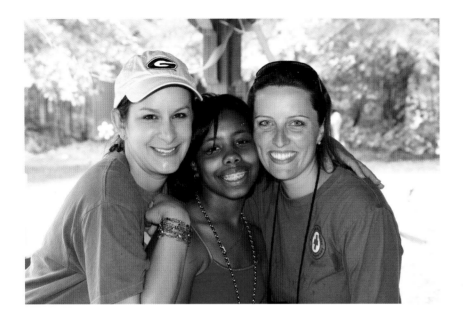

Dawn (left) with camper and fellow nurse

The ropes course is tucked away at camp, off the beaten path. That is one of the coolest places because it is where you see a lot of amazing things happen. I was a ropes course activity counselor my first year. There are kids who are amputees and are climbing to the top, and it just wows you. I remember having a few of those moments. Just being awestruck, thinking *gosh, look at these kids*. They were kids that I had taken care of. That was humbling for me my first year at camp. Being new

to a nursing career, I had not learned how to balance that toughness at work yet—figuring out boundaries for coping is important. I just remember that being such a bright spot of *wow. These kids go out and do things and are OK.*

I recall going back to work and taking care of a few of the kids that had gone to camp and being able to say, "Hey, I was at camp with you," or, "Hey, what fun it was." I felt like the kids look at you in a different way.

It makes nursing a little easier. Now they may be a little more willing to do what they need to do for you in the hospital because they see you as a real person. They know that you're there for a good reason and not just trying to do painful things to them, which sometimes is how it feels as a nurse. Camp gives you that little one up of "oh, she's my buddy. She was at camp. Yeah, I'll do this." That's kind of neat too.

I think about the catchphrase, "a ray of light," and that is what camp is. I've seen so many kids go through what they do in their cancer treatment, and you talk to them about Camp Sunshine. Most of the time, at first, they are not super excited about it. Most of the time you have to talk them into it that first year. Once they do camp, then they become ambassadors for those next kids and kind of bring that full circle. I love that piece of it. Being connected and being a part of that are special for me.

I think what has given me longevity as a nurse and volunteer is that the Camp Sunshine community gives you a reality check every day: *Don't sweat the small stuff, right?* Things could be worse. Camp gives you the ability to be thankful and feel blessed every day, which I think people in their busy lives tend to lose. I love that that is what camp gives me. Work does too, but Camp Sunshine does in a very special way.

One of the people who has meant a lot to me is Carrie Turner. I was Carrie's primary nurse in the hospital. I took care of her all throughout her AML journey. I fell in love with her and her family from the beginning. I remember early on sitting down with her mom and teaching her about leukemia and teaching them about what that means, how life is going to be different, and what you have to think about . . . learning counts and all these things that were so new to them. Her mom talks about that a lot now. She had a notebook, and she was taking all these notes. Later, she was so devastated when she lost the notebook because she had so many things that we had talked about written down. I remember telling her, "But you know all those things now. You didn't have to have them written down forever because you know them all. You learned them all. All those things became part of your journey."

I remember talking with Carrie about losing her hair. She was sixteen at the time. It is obviously very difficult to lose your hair as a teenage girl. I remember having that conversation with Carrie, and that is always a hard conversation. You can't minimize it because it is devastating. Sometimes that is the most devastating piece to a teenage girl. It was maybe around a prom or homecoming or not too long after. Carrie's hair was still really short, but she looked beautiful. She just rocked it. I loved seeing her on that special occasion—when she had been, at first, so vulnerable about losing her hair and thinking, "What am I going to look like?" Then, she was gorgeous in her new look. That was a neat, full-circle peace.

I had a special connection early on with Carrie and her family. The AML therapy is so hard. Seeing Carrie go through what she did in the hospital, and now she is a nurse and an adult—that is why I do what I do. You could not do it unless you had that peace to know that you made a difference and that that child went on and did great things like Carrie is doing. She has shared each step of the journey with me. I just love Carrie. She is the best. I loved being her primary nurse and seeing her throughout it all. Then, to have the opportunity to be with her at camp and to watch her grow and spread her adult wings is a real privilege.

I was so excited when Carrie told me, "I got into nursing school." I was so proud of her for so many little things along the way. Then, her reporting that she got a job—I have loved having those victories with her. It has just been so heartwarming. I think back, every time, to how sick she was and what she went through. I don't know that I could have done that at that age. She just picked herself up and kept on going and said, "You

know what? I'm going make a difference. I am going into the field that I was on the other side of to make a difference too."

Carrie is strong, first and foremost. She's driven, compassionate, sweet, and fun. And she is brave. It is important to me to maintain my relationship with Carrie because she still has so much of her journey left. The journey is her life and how she takes what she went through and uses that to make a difference. I remember having those conversations with her, "This is going to make you stronger. This is going to make you better," when she would be down and struggling. I truly believed that. I have seen so many kids go through it, and they do things that they may not have ever done had they not had cancer. I want to see what else Carrie does. I want to see her continue to grow into this amazing nurse, which I know she already is.

She has come full circle, now in her own career and seeing her own patients. I know what that means to her. Our relationship is a twofold thing: First, I watched her grow, and now, she is a fellow nurse. I'll always be protective of Carrie, her career, and what she wants to do. I would love to continue to be a mentor for her. She knows that I will always be there for her.

For as long as I am a pediatric oncology nurse, I need Camp Sunshine. I need camp for that grounding factor it has on my life. Camp is family. You don't ever think about severing ties with family. That is something you nurture, an important thing in your life that you put time into and grow.

What makes camp so special is intangible. At the heart of it is the circumstances that have brought these kids together.

They just "get" what the other is experiencing, it just happens. It is not just the kids at Camp Sunshine, it's also those connections you have with other counselors that you have volunteered with for years. You may not even see them throughout the year, but when you do, you just pick right back up. When you put all that together, it is magical.

10

Like a circle

Molly Casey (born August 22, 1966; hometown: Covington, Georgia)
and Hamilton Jordan, as told by Dorothy Jordan

MOLLY

People who ask me about being a childhood cancer survivor always ask if I was afraid of dying. I tell them I don't remember having that fear. I liked to play soccer as a young girl. I remember I woke up one morning after playing and my right leg was sore. I had a limp, and something was definitely wrong with my right knee.

My mother took me to the pediatrician, where I was prescribed antibiotics and blood thinner medication, but the pain persisted. I was taken to what was then DeKalb General Hospital, where a biopsy revealed that I had Ewing's sarcoma. I had a tumor about the size of an orange behind my right knee. The cancer had metastasized to both my lungs and sternum. My medical team wanted to do an amputation of my leg. I don't remember them discussing it with me—it was more of

a discussion with my parents. Because the cancer had metastasized, the doctors didn't give me very long to live. At the time, in 1980, with a diagnosis of metastatic Ewing's sarcoma, they were thinking I maybe had six months to live. I was thirteen years old.

Because the cancer had spread and because of the apparent limitation of time left for my life, my parents decided not to do the amputation. If I wasn't going to live very long anyway, why put me through the amputation? So after completing a second biopsy, my medical team devised an alternate treatment protocol for me, a combination of radiation and chemotherapy. We were going to fight this thing!

There were complications early on. My leg blocked up; I couldn't walk on it anymore. It was becoming useless to me. Because of the radiation, I developed an open wound that became infected. I could not fight the infection because of the chemotherapy and what it was doing to my immune system. And the cancer itself just kept spreading. Eventually my doctors could not tell what the tumor was versus what was the infection or what was causing what.

Again, my medical team raised the possibility of amputating my leg. This time it was different. This time they asked me what I wanted to do. They included me in the discussions. They said, "We could save you if we amputate the leg." I couldn't walk on it anymore. But on the positive side, I was having some success with the treatment protocol. The metastases were gone. The cancer remained only in my leg. So, as a freshman in high school in November 1981, I told the doctors to go forward with the amputation.

It didn't exactly work the way I had expected. I remember my mom saying, "They are still going to have to do chemotherapy, and you will still have to get through all that goes with it. But that's the point . . . you *will* get through this." And after another year and a half of treatment, I did.

I had just started high school, and my life was lonely. Basically, at school I wasn't around much as a freshman or sophomore. Because I had to go for blood tests two days a week, I missed so much time that I was sent back to make up classes. But I was fortunate to have my siblings. I have three brothers and a sister, and they wouldn't let me get away with anything. They didn't treat me any differently from how they treated each other, and they would not let me spend time feeling sorry for myself. They helped me become very independent, and I am so grateful for that and for all the support they gave me.

I remember getting fitted for my first prosthesis. The foam covering was wrapped in hosiery material to match the color of my real leg. I was uncomfortable, especially in the summertime, and every time I wore it, I couldn't wait to take it off. I had lost my hair during chemotherapy, and I remember the wig and the leg coming off as soon as I got home from school. But I was concerned about my physical looks. I wore the leg to school because I didn't want to use crutches. With crutches I couldn't carry anything, not even my books. So I learned to walk with my prosthesis. As uncomfortable and awkward as the artificial leg was, I persevered with it.

Sally Hale, my pediatric oncology nurse at the cancer clinic, and my oncologist Dr. Ragab told me about a plan to start a summer camp for children with cancer. I got to be an original Camp Sunshine camper. I was there the very first year. I was excited because I had never been to a camp before, but that meant I was

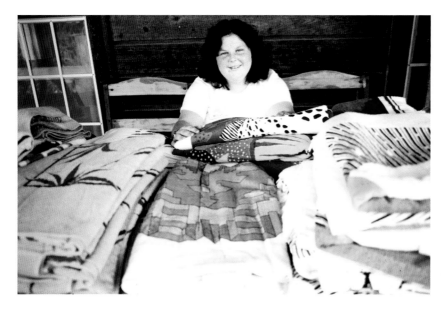

*Molly in 1983 at the first
Camp Sunshine*

scared, too, because I had never been to a camp before. I was nervous about my mobility and my prosthetic leg. But upon arriving at camp, I was greeted by Camp Sunshine founder Dorothy Jordan. Dorothy was right there to welcome me, and she just made me feel so good about being there. She asked me to help with checking people in. And that was that. I felt at home.

At the cancer clinic, you're just so sick. You just don't feel like chatting with folks. You're not necessarily thinking about making friends; you're mostly just thinking about not throwing up. At the hospital, in the days before there was a cancer center at Children's Healthcare of Atlanta, you were probably in a private room and isolated. And if you did do activities, you weren't necessarily with kids who had cancer. So that first camp was awesome. It was just like being with any other group of kids, except at Camp Sunshine, unlike at school or anywhere else, I did not have to worry about what I looked like or what I could or couldn't do. I had no qualms about being there. At the end of the day, it was just a bunch of kids you knew who cared about each other and wanted to have fun together.

Before cancer I had been a swimmer. I had not been swimming since my amputation. Camp got me back in the water. I joined the swim team, and I can clearly remember swimming in the lake. The activities we did at that first camp week were very basic: water games, a talent show, arts and crafts where we made the silliest things out of the silliest things. One of my fondest memories of that first camp was doing archery because I had never done it before. I thought, *Here is something new I can do even if I have cancer.* It was empowering.

I remember Hamilton Jordan's kindness and encouraging spirit during those early days of camp. I had no idea about his background, his service as chief of staff during Pres. Jimmy Carter's administration, any of that. To me, he was just Hamilton. He was just another goofy counselor that everybody loved.

Hamilton was just a big kid at heart. He wanted to play all the games with us; he wanted to jump in the lake with us. Whether I was on crutches or wearing that stupid leg, Hamilton was always encouraging me to try things I had never tried before. He told me it was ok to be afraid to do something new, but it wasn't ok not to try.

Hamilton was always so kind and good to us. After camp ended, Hamilton contacted me and my family. He had tickets to a Michael Jackson concert in Tennessee. That was my first concert, and I will never forget it. Hamilton made us feel so special, yet normal. Having that kind of role model at that time was an incredible gift for me.

In 1990, I returned to camp as a volunteer. I had not been to camp for six years and was not sure what to expect. I was nervous, but as soon as I got there, it was like I had never left. It was just so welcoming. Everyone treated me as if we had been together yesterday and just like I had never been gone. That's Camp Sunshine. That's the way it is.

I was diagnosed again in 1997, this time with cancer of the jaw. Even that did not deter me from returning to camp. Today, I rejoice in having been a Camp Sunshine volunteer for twenty-five years and counting, with many of those years working as a cabin counselor for girls aged ten to twelve. Generally, cabin counselors have the same group of girls for three years, and we try to keep them together from year to year. That way they can form friendships and real bonds.

Sometimes my campers want to know some of my story and ask, "What happened to you?" But more often they ask questions about my mechanical leg because it's

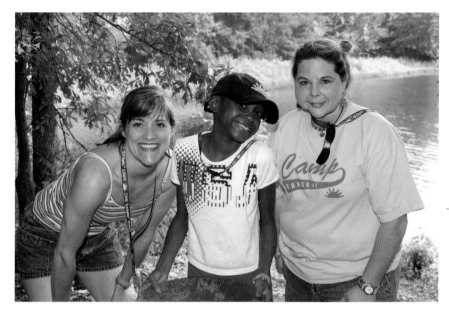

Molly (right) with fellow counselor and camper

cool for the kids to see and learn about it. My current prosthesis is a testament to the advances in prosthetics since my first artificial leg in the early 1980s.

Camp is like a family. You know, it's easy to lose perspective in day-to-day life. You can get caught up in so many things, so many details. Staying involved with camp helps me remember what is important, like not to sweat the small stuff and that people are good. There are many, many good people, amazing people in this world from all walks of life. Although we hear stories of kids today being spoiled, not appreciating what they have or behaving badly, I can tell you that 99.99 percent of the children I have met at Camp Sunshine are just good kids who want the chance to be normal. We all enjoy letting them do that.

I've had the satisfaction of seeing Camp Sunshine programs expand through the years. If a kid is a little nervous about going to Camp Sunshine for a week,

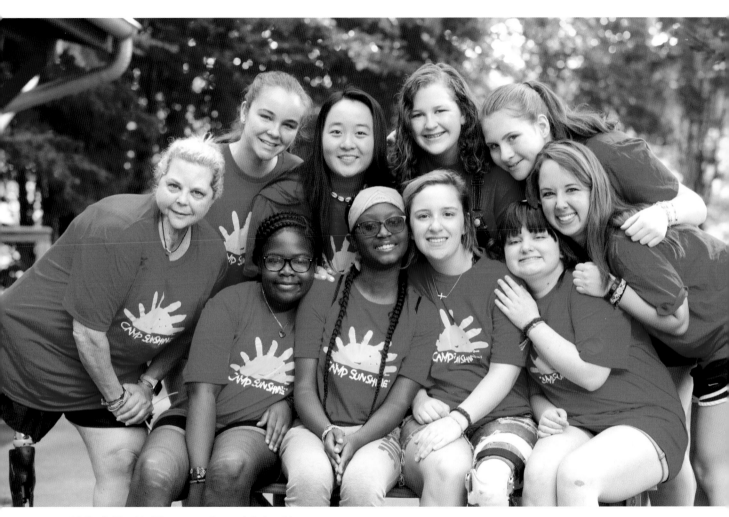

Molly (left) with fellow counselor and their cabin

at least they can try a day program or family weekend first. That way they get to know some people and it won't be so scary to go to summer camp. Those activities are also helpful for the parents. My own parents divorced in the years following my cancer. They didn't have the kind of support system that camp offers now. I think that would have been beneficial for my family. I truly appreciate that camp has these kinds of programs for the whole family now.

The Camp Sunshine community is like a circle. Hamilton was there for me when I had cancer, and I was there for him years later when he was battling his own cancer. I was working at Piedmont Hospital, where he was receiving treatment. Every time he was there, we would make it a point to see each other—just to check in on how we were both doing. I was very, very upset when he passed away. I cannot exactly put my finger on why he had such an impact on me as a child, but you can't explain camp. You can't explain the people. I can't explain the effect camp has had on me, not even to my own family. Sally Hale called me the day Hamilton died. She said Dorothy, his wife, wanted me to know before I heard it on the news. These people are so important to me; it is truly hard to explain.

Camp is something people have to experience for themselves. In all my years with Camp Sunshine, I have never heard anyone say they regretted having gone to camp. There was a camper last summer who was so homesick that she cried Sunday night and all day Monday. Her counselors tried everything to make her feel comfortable, but they finally called her parents to pick her up. That night as her cabinmates and counselors were discussing the next day's activities, the camper had a change of heart and decided to stay after all. She stayed the rest of the week and cried again—but this time it was when it was time to leave!

Without Camp Sunshine, I think I would have been much more afraid to try things or do things. I think I'm a much more confident person because of camp. Tricia, Sally, Hamilton and Dorothy, and the Dobies: these people were all about building the self-confidence we needed as kids. It was not easy being a teenager and having cancer and being so different from other teenagers, but at Camp Sunshine, none of that mattered.

I have worked at Piedmont Hospital for thirty years now as an IT specialist. I have five nieces, three nephews, and one great-nephew, all of whom I adore. I have had a busy life, but Camp Sunshine is as important to me today as it ever has been, although for different reasons. When I was a teenager and fighting cancer, camp was important because it was a chance for me to be independent of my family, to learn to connect with others, to have fun, and to grow. Now it's important because it *is* family. As an adult, I can give back to camp for all I have gotten from it. One of the great things about camp is having all the survivors who continue on as volunteers. It's important for the kids to see that continuum.

For me, camp is a time to reconnect with myself, to refocus myself and my priorities. Camp helps me understand all of the little things that are not important and all of the big things that are. I tell people that one reason I go back to camp every year is to get recharged.

Even my family doesn't really understand my connection to camp. It's love; it's friendship. I can say all these words, but I still cannot describe the feeling I get as I pull down the road to camp and see the Camp Sunshine logo. It's home. And it's a shame that not everyone gets to go.

Hamilton died on May 20, 2008, at age sixty-four, after twenty-three years of fighting his own battles with multiple cancers. I can't begin to tell you what Hamilton would say about Molly. I think he would express his immense love for her, and I can picture him

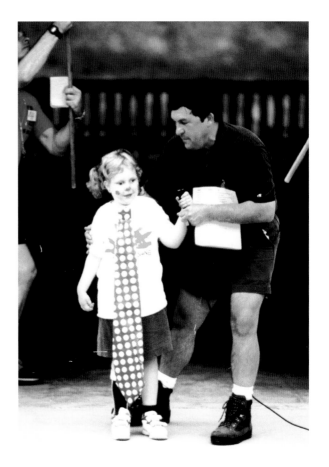

Hamilton, MC at camp talent show

shaking his head as he spoke of all that cancer had dealt Molly, smiling with pride at her courage and resilience. Vividly, I can picture both my first memory and my last memory of Hamilton and Molly together.

In 1983, standing on the camp dock on Lake Burton in north Georgia, in an untucked wrinkled blue dress shirt, faded blue gym shorts, with loosely tied running shoes, no socks, an athletic build, thick black hair and ruddy complexion, Hamilton is joking with thirteen-year-old Molly. With her freckled face, thick head of curly brown hair, bathing suit and shorts, she is sitting on the dock, her leg tucked up underneath her, her prosthesis thrown across the dock. Hamilton is devising a plan to get Molly back into the water, back to the sport she loved—swimming. He's making his case that you don't need two legs to swim. Molly's trust and then amusement is evident. The next scene in my mind is shrieks of surprise at the lake's cold temperature and then laughter. I see Mo Thrash, another volunteer who loved fun and pranks as much as Hamilton, there too, supporting Molly as she slid back into what was a safe, comforting place for her, the water.

Fast forward to 2008, I am wheeling Hamilton through the bottom floor of Piedmont Hospital in Atlanta. Hamilton was intent on finding Molly, now an IT specialist at the hospital. They had this unspoken connection, and the direction of support had changed. Hamilton is there for his umpteenth peritoneal draining, a procedure that requires use of ultrasound, necessary two to three times a week to remove the liters of fluid accumulating in his abdomen related to this last of several malignant diagnoses, this time mesothelioma. Hamilton is relieved to see Molly, a beautiful smile on her strong, lovely face. She leans into Hamilton in his wheelchair to hug him; Hamilton adjusts his oxygen tubing, removes the pulse oximeter from his finger, and runs his fingers through his still dark, not quite as thick hair, and cracks a joke. Now, his face is pale and thin, and his eyes are mostly sad, but they suddenly flash with a hint of his "smartass" humor and his love and pride for Molly. In Molly's preceding comments, she talks about the *circle of camp* and the evidence of that full circle of connection and caring is right here in front of me. With Molly's strength and composure, her resilience and courage in clear view, it was her turn to pass it back to Hamilton now for him to glean even a morsel of it, just to get him through the hour, then the day.

In his book about his own life and early cancer experiences, *No Such Thing as a Bad Day* (2000), Hamilton wrote: "*It was at Camp Sunshine that I really learned about cancer and the enduring lessons of life. . . . Camp*

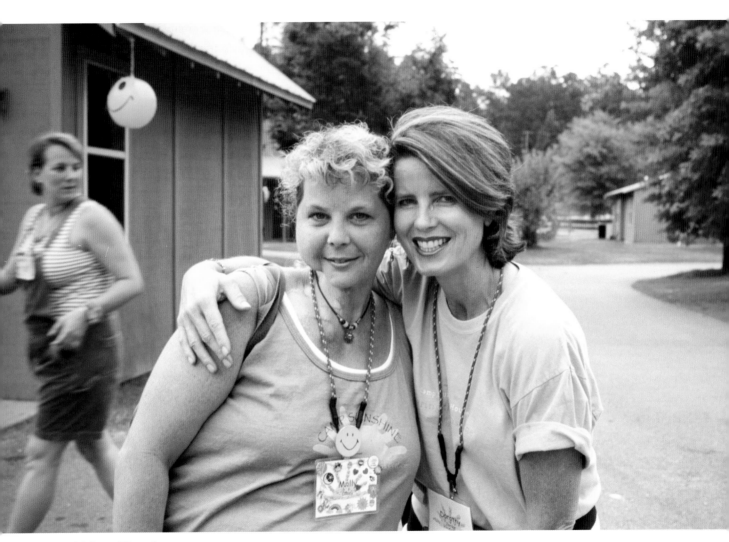

Molly and Dorothy

Sunshine has had a major impact on our lives, especially by giving us the opportunity to witness time and time again dramatic demonstrations of the power of the mind and attitude to alter the course of disease."

Hamilton told about the impact of the lives and stories, *"of the brave [Camp Sunshine] children who have touched our lives in so many ways. They have taught us to live and sometimes have shown us how to die."*

In the final chapter of his book, Hamilton wrote, *"For reasons I have never been able to understand, people with cancer are a remarkable group of brave, unselfish, and caring people. Maybe these people are changed forever by coming in touch with their own mortality, because the cancer patients I have known and cared about over the years are a remarkable group of human beings with a great spirit and a zest for living."*

Molly exemplifies the great spirit that Hamilton wrote about and Hamilton did too. Their lives were fuller because of the decades-long bond they formed, made possible by Camp Sunshine, and I am so grateful.

Hair and limbs are optional

Kati Tanner Gardner (born September 8, 1980; hometown: Woodstock, Georgia)
and Dr. Roger Vega

KATI

I was at a Halloween party at my daycare in 1988 and was dressed as Cleopatra. It was the first time my mom had ever bought me a nongrocery store costume. She went to the costume store and bought me a costume. I had to beg to go to the party. My aunt took me because my little sister was getting an ear infection. I was wearing sneakers, and it had rained, because it rained every Halloween. I walked in. I turned to talk to one friend, and I turned back around.

As I was turning back around my feet just flew out from under me, and I snapped my femur. I heard it pop and felt something. I'd just walked into this party that I had been begging to go to, and I said, "That's it, I want to go home" because it hurt. I couldn't put any pressure on my leg at all. My aunt questioned, "Are you

sure? You don't want to go play this game?" I was adamant, "No, I just want to go home." My aunt took me home, and my parents asked what had happened. They thought that maybe I had dislocated my hip or something because I still couldn't move my knee. My dad got my favorite sweat suit because it was the '80s and we wore sweat suits a lot back then.

My parents took me to the local ER. There, the doctors basically looked at me and said, "No, she broke her femur. This is what happens. This is how it works." They took me back, and they cut my favorite sweat suit off of me. I was so devastated. They did the X-rays, and sure enough, I had snapped my femur in half. The doctor that was on call told my parents, "Listen, I see a little cyst, but I'm not going to biopsy it because I see these in kids all the time. It's nothing." He then proceeded to sedate me and put a pin through my shin because the way they set femurs back then was in traction, so I was in traction for three and a half weeks in the hospital. We were under the impression that in three and a half, four weeks, whatever, I would be fine.

I started running a low-grade temperature in the hospital, but nobody thought much of it. I was released on Thanksgiving Day in a brace. Usually, they would put kids in those Spica casts that separated their legs, and that's what they were in for a while at home. Then they would just cut it off, and they would go about life, but they thought I was a good candidate for this brace so I could slowly get mobility back. Not until around Christmas was I able to start sitting up.

In January, I started being able to bend my knee. I went back to school. I hadn't been to school since Halloween. Things were going fine, and then, around Presidents' Day weekend in February, I started feeling really crappy. I didn't feel good. I didn't leave my bedroom. I had started noticing that every time I bent my knee, it hurt. I would feel something go up into my thigh and pop. It didn't hurt, it was just a really bad sensation, and I did not like it, so I just did not do anything.

That was a four-day weekend, and my mom got me up to go to school on Tuesday after me not leaving my bedroom and not eating much of anything that weekend. She tried to put the brace back on me, and it would not lace up. My leg had swollen. She called my dad in there, and they finally got the Velcro to go around. My mom tried to talk me out of going to school, but I was determined to go because it was picture day, and picture day to a second grader is a big deal. I was wearing this black sweatshirt that had neon curly-Q ribbons on it, and I loved it. My dad was going to pick me up early that day because I had physical therapy (PT). I had started PT at this point, and I hated my physical therapist. She was mean, and she wasn't used to working with kids, and it was terrible. This was not at our children's hospital.

The whole day at school was terrible, just terrible, terrible, terrible. My dad picked me up from school that day and took me to PT which was just above my surgeon's office. He said, "Listen, she is in a lot of pain, and there is a lot of swelling." My physical therapist at first dismissed it and remarked, "Well, she is whiny. She is just a whiner. She will just need to get over it. You are going to have to make her do this. She just doesn't want to do it." My dad replied, "Well, why don't we get an X-ray just to be safe because there's a lot of swelling."

Dad persisted. I remember sitting in the exam room with him, and the orthopedic surgeon that had previously told my parents it was just a cyst came in.

I remember I could see his beard had grown, and he had gotten so pale. He said, "I am referring you to Dr. Monson over at Crawford Long, and you have an appointment tomorrow morning. We want you there at 8:00 a.m. You need to be there at 8:00." That is all they told us. I found out later that when my dad called my mom and told her what was going on, she told her coworkers. She said, "Something is wrong, and I don't know when I'll be back." She realized this was not good.

We went the next day and met with Dr. Monson. He basically looked at my parents and said, "Your daughter has a huge tumor on her leg. It's encapsulating her femur." I remember it made my mom cry, and at that moment, I hated him for making my mom cry. Over the next two days, I had a CT scan, bone scan, and every test known to man.

It took a little while to get the diagnosis. At first, they thought I had osteosarcoma just based on numbers. They did my pathology twice and it came back finally as Ewing's sarcoma. I was eight, so the only thing I knew about Ewing's then, at that moment, was that maybe they could do a limb salvage. They had said if it was osteosarcoma they would amputate because back then the standard of care was to amputate before you even started chemo, but if it was Ewing's, they would give me a few rounds of treatment and see what happens.

When it came back as Ewing's sarcoma I thought, "OK, well, this just probably means I'll get to keep my leg."

Then we met Dr. Vega at Egleston. I remember him being very serious during our first meeting, which is odd because he is rarely ever serious with me now! I just remember that first meeting being very solemn. They randomized me, and I was put on a clinical trial. I did not get the standard of care at the time for Ewing's. I got the VP16 Ifosfamide protocol, which is now the standard of care, and my first treatment was the VP16 Ifosfamide combination for five days. During my treatment, I was inpatient. My treatment lasted eighteen months. I lost most of second and all of third grade.

We did three rounds of treatment, which took us to mid-April, early May. They rescanned me, and my parents met with Dr. Monson. My parents were always great about letting me be in the room with any conversations that I wanted to hear, but I remember, this one in particular, I said, "I don't want to be in this conversation." We didn't have child life specialists back then, and I remember having anxiety thinking about it. It just made me feel nervous to be in that conversation.

I sat in Dr. Monson's office, and I hung out with one of his technicians, somebody that I had just become friendly with. We played with clay and Play-Doh while my parents had this very important discussion.

Dr. Monson came back with, "Here are your options. We can try a limb salvage procedure, or we can do an amputation." He gave us the pros and cons with both. There were a lot of cons to me with this idea of the limb salvage procedure. I was going to need surgery every time I grew. I was going to have to have radiation. It was going to extend my treatments, and there was a good chance that my left leg would never grow the way my right leg did. It was a lot more surgery. I talked to my parents a lot about it. We bounced around ideas. I remember at one point saying, "Yeah, we'll do the limb salvage," and then within a couple hours I was saying, "No, hm-mmm. I don't want to do that."

My parents let me make the decision to amputate, even at eight. My mom was worried that I was going to come back to her at sixteen and say, "Why did you let this child make this decision?" I never regretted it. There were moments that it's inconvenienced me significantly, but I've always known that it saved my life.

On May 25, 1989, they did my amputation. It was twenty-nine years ago this past May. I celebrate it. I look at it as my happy birthday. I was mostly "pissed off" because I wasn't getting to go to Camp Sunshine the next week because camp was the first week of June. All of my friends that I had made while on chemo—Prisca, Ron, Sam, and Brian—we had all been diagnosed within weeks of each other. They were all getting to go to camp, and I wasn't, and, man, was I hot! My mom said, "You had your leg amputated three days ago. We are not sending you."

I had heard about camp before my amputation. Ann, my night nurse, was the first person to tell me about Camp Sunshine. It must have been during my first treatment, and she was telling my mom about how much fun campers had and what a great time it was. I think we all looked at her like she was a little bit cuckoo!

The next time I heard about Camp Sunshine was before my amputation, when I was at the signing for Erma Bombeck's book *I Want to Grow Hair, I Want to Grow Up, I Want to Go to Boise*. Sally Hale was in front of me in line, so I met Sally that day and she told me about camp too. Then I met Erma Bombeck. My mom had been reading me Erma's books at night before we even knew this book was coming out. Then this book came out right in the middle of when we needed it most. I still have my copy of it. I have a picture of me and Erma Bombeck at that signing. Those were the two instances that I heard about Camp Sunshine, but I had to wait a whole year before I got to go.

First, the buildup about camp was happening at the clinic, and then when everybody came home, I was so mad. Miss Sydney (therapeutic play person at the clinic) would play the videos of camp, of all of camp, because Mr. Sydney, a volunteer, had walked around with this VHS recorder all week. She would play them in the clinic. While we were waiting to go back for treatment, she would play all of these videos. I got to watch the talent show. I thought, *I'm going to this*. By the time I got to go to camp, I had been amputated for over a year, and I had two rounds of chemo left. I was still bald.

My first year at camp was 1990. We were at Camp Barney Medintz. I remember driving in and being super excited. When I walked into the gym, it just seemed like there were thousands of people there. My counselor Jane walked up to me and said, "You're Kati Tanner, aren't you?" I was, like, "Huh?" She gave me my first camp bracelet. I was in Cabin One, and Jane and Maryann were my counselors. Prisca and I were in the same cabin with Sarah and that was Sarah's first summer too.

I remember I danced at the talent show. The first day came around, and we were choosing our activities, and I saw dance. I said, "Oh, I can't go to that." My counselor Jane said, "Oh, yes, you can. Do you want to go to dance?" I said, "Well, I mean, yeah." I had done ballet like every little girl, but really, I was

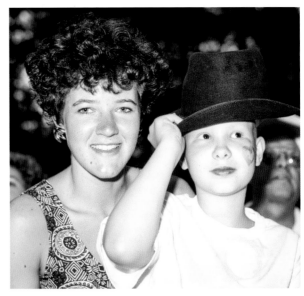

Kati, her first year at camp with counselor

just a ham. She replied, "OK, you are going to dance," so I went to dance. Lauren was the dance teacher. We danced to "Magic to Do" from *Pippin*, and Prisca and I started out on stage on either side. I was stage right. We came out at the beginning doing these fun little arm motions, and I thought, *This is the best place*. This, I believe, led to my theater major!

Besides dance, I remember doing karate with Karate Steve and Cindy helping me do a cartwheel in gymnastics. I have very, very vivid memories of camp. It rained some, but it didn't rain the whole week. I remember feeling like I never had to explain to anybody why I was bald. I didn't have to worry about whether people were going to think I was a boy or a girl.

It was a defining moment in my life, going to Camp Sunshine that summer. I did everything. I just did everything. Dixie was still around then, and she was doing really well. We had become little buddies. She would help me paint my crutches and things like that. I remember thinking also that she was just gorgeous and if I could look like her when I grew up life would be great. I'm sure she was around t̲hirteen, but in my head, she was a grown-up.

I was also able to go to one of the first family camps. That is where I met Dustin for the first time. He had just been diagnosed. Dustin was very progressive, and he had an earring even at ten. He walked by me, and he was bald, and I saw an earring. So, we just assumed girl. I walked up to him, "Hey, my name's Kati. What's your name?" He replied, "Dustin," and I said, "Oh!" It was the biggest shock. We discovered very quickly that we were both very naturally competitive. The fact that we were both amputees and we were the same age and we were amputated at same level, both being hip disarticulations, we became very competitive with each

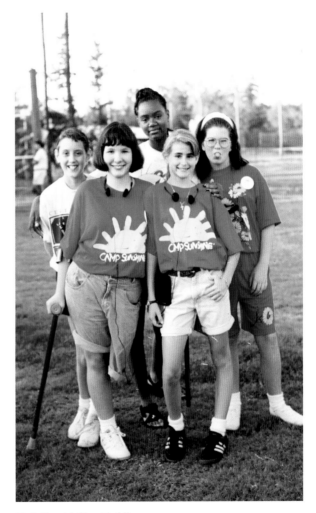

Kati (front left) with fellow campers

other almost instantly. The big difference was that he was much more naturally athletic than I was. There were things that he just totally smoked me at, but I was a little more adventurous than he was. I was much more outgoing, so there were other things that I totally smoked him at. Our families competed against each other at Family Feud at that first family weekend. My family got all of them right except one, and his family stole it, and I was so mad.

My core friends were my camp friends. My school friends were school friends, and they were great, but my core friends—if I had had a bad day and needed to vent, I was going to call Sarah or Talley or Jeff. I wasn't going to call somebody that I went to school with. A lot of times there was a maturity difference between my school friends and me. Especially by the time I got to high school because Dustin died in eighth grade. That was really hard. I remember just sitting there and feeling like I was going to come unglued at any moment. These typical fourteen-year-olds around me just did not and could not comprehend what I was feeling. In high school, people would be talking about who was with who and that type of thing, and I was like, y'all don't even know . . .

I spent a lot of time waiting for my friends to catch up. Plus, I lived life as a very obvious one-legged girl. I have never worn a prosthesis for any amount of time. I have never had a problem with that, but it does draw attention, wanted or unwanted. I never had that problem at camp. I have always said Camp Sunshine is a place where hair and limbs are optional. If your IV pole is your date to the dance, all the better.

There are so many favorite memories. There are the kind of girly ones that I feel like every kid should get to have, when the boy that likes you or that you like comes and sits next to you. That didn't happen in school for me, but it happened at camp. That was defining for me. I will never forget that Brett chose to sit next to me in the dining hall, and that was huge. We never were boyfriend and girlfriend, but it didn't matter because he chose to sit next to me, and that was amazing. I got three awards that have stuck out with me over the many years that I have been to camp. One was my very first award, and Jane gave me the Spirit of Camp Sunshine. I feel like it just set me on a trajectory for life.

When I was sixteen, Kim and Bubbles were my counselors. This was when we still did awards in front of everybody, and they would give a little explanation. Kim said, "If you know Kati, you'll understand this award," and they gave me the Leadership Award. I remember walking up to receive it. It is special that they acknowledged me that way even at that young of an age. Then, my last year as a camper, Bubbles and Stacy gave me the Big Heart Award. That was special. Those were all memorable moments.

Camp is home. It is my safe space. I took a seven-year hiatus when my little girls were born, with my last summer in 2008. I had dinner one night in 2015 with camp friends Mary Katherine and Sarah, and they said, "You should come back!" At that point I was wondering if maybe camp had moved on. I had been gone a long time. Maybe that chapter in my life was closed, and it hurt to think about that. I missed camp more than I ever missed my leg. It was like this person-shaped hole in my soul. I said, "OK, I'm going to come back next year. I'm going to do it."

So I went back in 2016. In April 2016, after I had sent in my forms to be a volunteer, my mom unexpectedly passed away. She just died in the middle of the night. It was terrible. I remember driving into camp, and it was hard because I didn't have her to call. I got out of the car, and Jackman (camp volunteer and friend) had gotten there at the same time. When Tenise called me Kati Tanner when I checked in, I was like, "I'm home." I mean, I was a grown-up, but it was home. As hard as it was, and it was really hard, that week healed me in a way I don't think I could have healed had I not gone to camp. The next year was difficult in general, but I

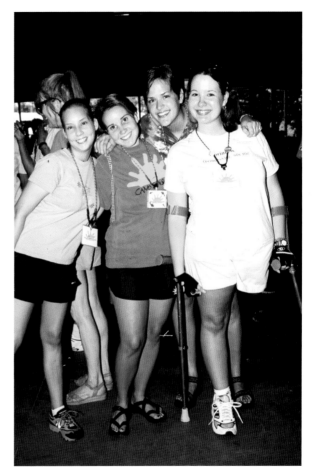

Kati (far right) at teen camp

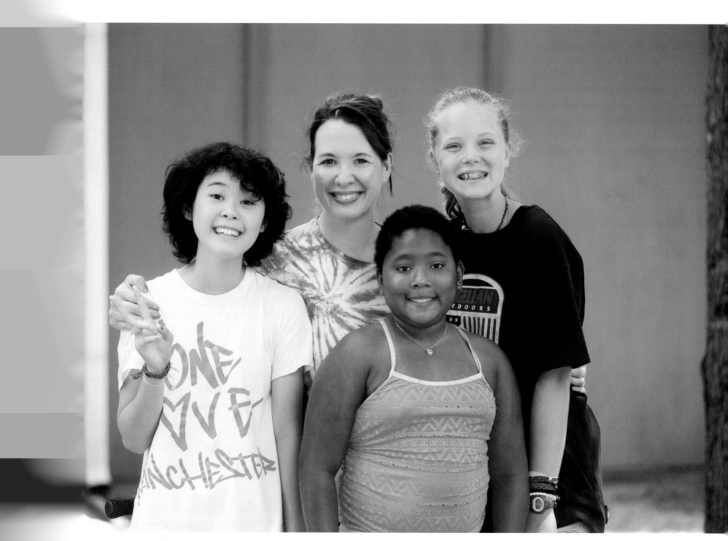

i as counselor with her campers

leaned into those moments at camp and remembered them.

When I did return in 2016, I was nervous. Did I still remember how to be a good camp counselor? My campers had all gotten there, and they were brand-new thirteen-year-olds, brand new to teen week, which is kind of my favorite. I had this camper, who had rotationplasty procedure (a type of amputation). We were walking together, and she said, "I'm really glad to have another one-legged person in my cabin so somebody can walk slow with me." I thought, *I will walk slow with you forever.* I thought, *This is why I come to camp. This is why I am here.* That camper is still in my cabin, three years later, and now she passes by me all the time. She is gone in an instant, and I remind her, "Don't you remember? We're supposed to walk slow together!"

The community of camp has meant everything to me. Camp Sunshine counselors attended my high school plays, even though I did not live close to Atlanta. They came to my graduation; they came to my graduation parties. They drove to see me in the Miss Brenau Pageant during my freshman year of college. Luckily, I won, so I made the journey worth their while!

For every monumental moment in my life since 1990, whether it was an off-therapy party, my Sweet Sixteen party, even my wedding, Camp Sunshine has been there. I remember thinking that my wedding was the best party ever because it had every sector of my life in one room.

People from camp have been integral to my story during different parts of my life. Bubbles helped me grow up. She helped me go from being a teenager to an adult. There is a big leap when you graduate from college, and I remember a lot of my friends floundered with it. They weren't sure how to go from being students to real grown-ups. She helped me bridge that gap. She also taught me a lot about advocating for myself. Once we were in a store in Little Five Points and somebody gave me a bag with no handles. Bubbles told me, "No, you need to go back, and you need to say, 'I really need a bag with handles.'" And she was right. Ever since then, every time I check out at a store, I say, "Oh, actually, can you please put that in a bag with handles?" or, "Can you separate that into two bags for me instead of putting everything in one?" Those are little life lessons that make me think of Bubbles every time.

Dr. Vega has always been there for me. Even now that he is retired, I could send him an email tomorrow and he would get back to me. I almost asked him to give me away at my wedding. Dr. Vega has always been that person. Even after he left Children's Healthcare of Atlanta (CHOA), I knew I could still go see him, and I did. I went to the long-term survivors' clinic at CHOA until I was too old. I remember taking my daughter Kennedy to my follow-up appointments.

When I found out that I was pregnant, I first told my husband, then we told my mom and next Dr. Vega. He immediately told me, "If you get too tired, if you can't breathe good, if you feel crappy, I want you to go to the emergency room and have them look at your heart."

That's when I found out that I had cardiomyopathy. Dr. Vega always empowered us as patients to know about our disease and to know what was going on and to know the potential side effects even as we became grown-ups. We were the first generation of survivors, so they are just now figuring out what is happening to us. Especially with Ewing's sarcoma, there is just not a large number of us.

I have been married now for eleven years. I met my husband doing a fundraiser for the Keencheefoonee Road Race (volunteer run for camp). He was a summer associate at the law firm where I was working. Now we have two girls. They are five and nine. Kennedy was born in 2009, and Eleanor was born February 28, 2013, which is almost twenty-five years to the day of my diagnosis at the very same hospital. I look at it as, they have taken one leg away, but they gave me two more back.

Now I am a writer. I have been very blessed. I have worked hard. I have worked really hard. I want to keep writing books about teenagers with chronic illness and disability but where nobody dies, where they are living with it and it is not about tragedy, but empowerment. I want to keep writing those books. I want to go into schools and talk a lot about identity and how it is OK to be disabled. That doesn't mean I am different. It just means I am disabled. You are abled, and I am disabled. They are not bad words.

I get frustrated when I hear parents say, "Well, I don't want them to grow up thinking they are disabled." They are disabled. That is fine. It is like saying I have brown hair. I want to talk a lot about that. I talk a lot about using pieces from your story in your life. I wrote *Brave Enough*. In it, Cason has Ewing's sarcoma, and she ends up an amputee. That is the beginning and end of how we are similar, but that is a part of me as well. She goes to cancer camp. That is a big part of me.

Camp is still home. It is still what I use to mark my years. I don't mark the beginning of my year January 1. It is the week I go to camp. It is for when I set New Year's resolutions. Camp is always my touchstone. I feel like I can never give enough to Camp Sunshine to reap half of what it has given me and continues to give me by letting me hang out with these teenagers for a week, listen to them talk, and to maybe every now and then be able to throw in a piece of advice. I can never give back what it has given to me.

Camp is family, and it's the family that never judges me. It is not the family I am ever embarrassed by. When life gets too crazy, and it does, I always know that I can come back to camp.

I want to tell kids who are first being introduced to Camp Sunshine that they will be safe and loved, no matter what is going on in life. Sometimes a camper's cancer is the least of what they are managing. No matter what they are facing this week, I want to tell them, *I will keep you safe, and I will love you.*

I wrote about Camp Sunshine in my book, *Brave Enough.* In the book, somebody asks Mari, who is a camper, if she could live anywhere in the world, where would she live. She says, "I would live here, but I would have to keep all of these people here with me." Camp is the people. There is that verse in the Bible that says wherever two or more are gathered, there is church. I feel that way about camp. Wherever there are two of us, we are at camp. That is what it is. It is the people. The space is glorious, and we are so lucky to have it. If you take us out of it, it is just a place. I don't know what

magic was sprinkled to make that happen, but that is why I have gone for twenty-two years. That is why I have been there from 1990 and can remember names and faces and stories.

There are campers and counselors that we have lost over the years. They are still present; we still feel and see them. Yesterday, it was Dustin Dove's birthday, and I got to sing him happy birthday while I was at camp, and that is special. If I can help people remember and tell their stories, I will.

ROGER

My wife, Ketty, and I came to New York from Puerto Rico to finish our training in pediatrics. We were recruited to work at St. Luke's Hospital, an affiliate of Columbia University. At that time, I had very little exposure to hematology-oncology. Columbia required three months of hematology-oncology training, and I had zero. After completing my training in pediatrics, I applied to a fellowship in pediatric oncology-hematology at Cornell-Memorial Sloan Kettering Cancer Center. I realized early in my fellowship that this was my calling and that I had a very strong connection with it.

As a resident physician in the hematology-oncology unit at Columbia, I met a little girl from New England, a patient who had a benign brain tumor. She was hospitalized and was going to have surgery, and she required a spinal tap every single day. Her parents were prominent people, affluent, and it was kind of understood that none of the resident physicians could talk to the girl or to the parents. They wanted only to talk to the attending doctor.

The weekend prior to her surgery, I was the resident on call, and I was going to have to do the spinal tap. I met the family on Friday, and I was to do the spinal tap on Saturday and Sunday. On Saturday I went into the little girl's room and spoke to her. I told her I saw how the doctor had done the procedure, but I thought I had a way to make it less painful. I also asked her parents, if they wouldn't mind, to leave the room while we did the spinal tap. I explained to all of them that the child was going to help me and that she was going to be a part of this procedure. They all agreed to let me do this.

I gave her a little anesthesia at the injection site to give her some numbness. And I kept talking and talking to her. I kept asking her questions about her family, her likes, her dislikes. I introduced the needle into the spine, and we just kept talking and talking. I pulled out the needle and said, we are done. She said, that can't be it. But yes, we were done. Her parents came back in the room, and she told them she hadn't felt a thing.

I repeated the procedure the next day and when the attending physician returned on Monday, he called me aside and commended me for a job well done. The little girl went into surgery on Wednesday; her tumor was benign and was removed. She was cured. I went to see her while she was recovering in the ICU, and I have never forgotten what she said to me. "You have to promise me something . . . you have to promise me that you'll study something that helps children like me . . . children who are sick, so they won't feel the pain." That's what did it. That's what set my career path.

It was Dr. (Abdel) Ragab who asked me if I would move to Atlanta and help start the bone marrow transplant program at Egleston Children's Hospital at Emory University. The year was 1984. Camp Sunshine had started in 1983, in the mountains of north Georgia. I had heard about these camp experiences for children when I was in New York, but it was still a relatively new idea. My curiosity was killing me. A summer camp for children who have cancer? How can this be? How can they do it? In 1985, I volunteered to go to camp. I think Dr. Ragab was very happy that I wanted to go. I went for the first time in 1985 and every year through 1999. Two weeks out of every year, I spent at camp, and the last seven or eight years, I was the medical director at Camp Sunshine. I loved it. It was an honor to be so involved with camp.

I had spoken to the nurses who had done the first two camps, and they were very enthusiastic about the benefits that camp had for these kids. The nurses told me that Camp Sunshine was absolutely phenomenal, that the kids had a wonderful time. But they also told me you have to be there for them, and I get that. Kids with cancer, their medical conditions can change so quickly. The medical care was an essential piece of camp.

My first time at Camp Sunshine, I was like a sponge. I wanted to learn everything I could . . . what could these kids do, and what couldn't they do, and what could we help them do, if they wanted to do it. It all depended on their (blood) counts. If their platelets were low, well, maybe no jumping or climbing or horsing around that day. But that didn't mean there weren't other things they could do. From the very beginning, camp was better than I expected it could be. I thought the kids might be moping around or feeling sad. Nothing could be further from the truth. They forgot they had cancer; they forgot they had limitations. They just grabbed the lion by the tail and just went for it!

With all the years I have worked in pediatric oncology, I have seen how these young patients can feed off

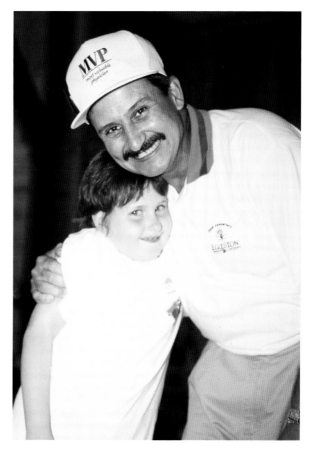

Dr. Roger Vega with camper

each other, support each other, and help each other. For example, the fears of one child can be quieted by the assurances of other children. We have kids who are on-therapy and kids who are off-therapy. At camp, we have kids who are newly diagnosed and kids who are cancer-free. And they all talk to each other. They all share with each other; they help each other; and they answer each other's questions. What kind of cancer do you have? ALL? That's what I have too. And maybe one kid who is bald-headed and filled with uncertainty can talk to another one who is doing fine and has a head full of hair. At camp, they can talk to each other with no judgments. They understand what each other are going through. They are speaking the same language. And that can be energizing.

Over the years, some things have changed, like the facilities. Camp today is at Camp Twin Lakes, which was built with input from the physicians. It is a facility that serves the physicians, the nurses, all the volunteers, and the campers well, extremely well. It is a superb and elaborate camp.

Some things might not happen today at camp that happened in the early days. For example, one night I came back from being out all day at camp, and I found a canoe in my room! After running around like a maniac all day being very busy and having fun with these kids, I come back to my room and I find a sixteen-foot canoe in my room. I can still see myself on that day. I mean, how did they get it in there? And now I had to find somebody to help me pull that sucker out! Those are the things you never forget about camp.

Camp was, and still is, a beautiful, beautiful experience. What has never changed is the commitment of the people who serve at Camp Sunshine . . . the volunteers, the nurses, and the staff. There are the nurses and the Sally Hales of the world who are just wonderful, wonderful people. And others who come to serve from lives and jobs not at all related to medicine or hospitals. In many cases these people are using their own time off from their job to be at Camp Sunshine—to be with children who have cancer so that these kids can have a week at camp, a week to be a kid again. That same spirit I saw thirty or more years ago at camp is still alive and present today. The way that camp changes the lives of kids, that is something that has not changed. I can't tell you how many times I have heard campers say to each other, "I can't wait until next year." They live from camp to camp, and this is a testament to the work that all of these people do at camp to make it such an extraordinary experience.

I have been a child at heart all my life—just ask my patients! I would rather be joking with them and laughing with them than always doing the serious doctor thing with them. Cancer is a very serious thing, but it doesn't have to be all serious business all the time, and that was the beauty of camp. I didn't have to always be a doctor. I could just be another crazy person at camp, running around and having a lot of fun with these kids.

I still have what I consider to be very, very good friends among the staff and volunteers at Camp Sunshine. The nurses who worked with me at camp and at the clinic, we share a special connection. Working together at camp and being with these children in a setting outside the clinic or the hospital setting, it just took our professional lives to the next level.

Kati Tanner Gardner is like family to me, and her family is like family. I used to go fishing with her father; the day her mother died, I was there with them. The connection I had with Kati and her family started in the hospital when Kati was very young and very sick, and it just continued and grew stronger at camp.

Kati is simply an unbelievable woman. She was so determined; I don't think I had ever seen anyone as determined as she was even as a child. Even as a young girl, Kati was in many long discussions about her treatment options, including whether or not she would need an amputation. I can remember her talking to

Dr. Monson and asking him where—what part of her leg—would be best to do the surgery . . . for the best outcome. He said the leg would be taken from the hip. Kati said, "Take it. It will be done." So it was. She was unbelievably strong and focused, and that determination of hers has always stayed with me. She was resilient too. She knew she would somehow get through this; she knew she would move on with her life. She was the same way when it came to her prosthesis too. I can remember her having a lot of trouble with her prosthesis. It never seemed to work right for her. Finally, she said, "I don't care—I just won't wear it anymore." That is Kati. She likes to move on and just go, go, go. Once she has made up her mind, there is no stopping her.

You know, nothing makes me happier than when I'm proven wrong . . . when I have had a young patient who grows up to be a young woman who marries and becomes pregnant. That is a very special time for me. I love to be proven wrong because, years ago as a pediatric oncologist, one thing we would talk to our young patients about was the fact that with all their treatment, all the chemotherapy, and such, they might not be able to have children. So I am absolutely thrilled when they contact me to tell me I was wrong! Kati's daughters are precious; they are little pistols. I guess they get that from their mother.

12 You can still climb this wall

Javier (Javi) Medina (born September 17, 1975; hometown: Riverdale, Georgia)
and Patty Miller

JAVIER

At the time of my diagnosis, I was fourteen years old. I was in the eighth grade at Pointe South Junior High in Riverdale, Georgia. I was playing basketball that season, but the sport I loved and excelled at was baseball. I also liked participating in neighborhood football games, playing Nintendo, and riding bikes through wooden trails with my friends. And believe it or not, this athletic, thrill-seeking kid was one of best violin players in the school. I was the only eighth grader in the Clayton County Youth Symphony, which was comprised of high school students. Then, of course, when my diagnosis happened, everything just paused and went south, and it wasn't the same again.

Basketball began in November. Tryouts and practices were every night. After running hard and trying our best to impress the coach for two straight hours, we were spent, sweaty, and hot. I remember coming out into the cool night air with nothing more on than a T-shirt and gym shorts—the hubris of a teenager. I had developed a limp; the source of the discomfort was my right hip. Since I was playing basketball, no one gave it a second thought. Maybe I pulled something while running suicides or sprinting down the court. But the limp didn't go away.

My parents took me to various sports medicine specialists who each performed their share of X-rays and evaluations. No muscle was pulled, no ligament or tendon was torn, and no bone was fractured or broken. I recall getting angry and frustrated at my parents because I knew something was wrong and no one was able to provide me any answers. I was missing school for the first time, after having perfect attendance from kindergarten. The straw that broke the camel's back was a Christmas shopping trip to the mall with my mom when I just was really lethargic and pale as a ghost. So, on December 16, 1989, my parents took me to a pediatrician. My doctor ordered blood work, and when she returned with the results, her teary-eyed expression told the whole story. I had a high volume of immature white blood cells that were causing my symptoms, including an infection in my hip that made me limp. The pediatrician told my parents to take me straight to Scottish Rite Children's Hospital, and the next day, a bone marrow test confirmed leukemia.

I was diagnosed with acute lymphoblastic leukemia (ALL). My mom cried. My father was stoic, but years later when I was in the clear, he confessed that he resented God. What got him was seeing the little kids in the hospital. A couple of them had bandages over their heads from brain surgery, and their little faces were swollen. That got him to question, "How can something like this happen to these little kids?" My youngest brother, Rob, who was six at the time, was a quiet kid and had a closer relationship with my middle brother, Luis, who was ten. I never saw Rob's or Luis's initial reaction to the news. We never had any conversation about my diagnosis, but never once did they express any sadness or fear.

My routine after a long and challenging morning at the oncology clinic was to spend the rest of the day dozing in my room. One of my most vivid memories is of my brothers coming home from school, cracking open my bedroom door, and poking their heads in just enough to see me. Then they asked my mom how the day went. My cancer fight matured them at a young age. I don't think they resented me for getting all the attention—they just knew I was sick, and that MaPa's (our parents' nickname) time and energy needed to be on me. Years later, my dad told me that my brother Luis said he wished he had cancer instead of me.

My girlfriend didn't know how to handle what was going on with me. Can anyone expect any teenager to know? I guess, at that time, not a lot of people knew about cancer. When I finally got back to school, kids thought I was contagious! I couldn't get mad at them because how else could teenagers react to something that they have never experienced before? So to make it easier on my girlfriend, I broke it off. I just wanted her life to go on without her worrying about me. Even after the breakup, she was still one of my first friends to visit me at home. She even baked me some cookies. I felt like a million bucks that day. Today, she is a staff nurse at Children's Healthcare of Atlanta.

Bactrim, prednisone, vincristine, methotrexate, Adriamycin, Cytoxan, l-asparaginase, 6-MP, spinal taps, bone marrow tests, and radiation—that was the cast of characters that dominated my first year of treatment. Frequency varied; sometimes it was once a week, sometimes every other day. Cranial radiation lasted about two weeks. During my last two years of treatment, I went to clinic once a month and visited with my old friend, vincristine. I sincerely say friend because it didn't give me any short- or long-term side effects. But for that first year, it seemed like I was hooked up to something every day.

Year one was not without its nasty curveballs. Although the only surgery I had was for my central line, that initial hospital visit would soon be the first of many. I was released just days before Christmas. Ma-Pa's main worry was my food and fluid intake. Doctors and nurses encouraged them to give me whatever I was in the mood for because the prednisone would take care of my appetite. And so they did. My parents were happy to give me whatever Christmas dessert and fruit juice I wanted. They saw this as a good sign, knowing the chemo's appetite-suppressing trademark.

My eating and drinking habits stayed the same after Christmas, but I felt lethargic, I was always thirsty, and frequent trips to the bathroom kept me up all night. Days before the New Year, I was scheduled for my next chemo session. The doctors did a complete blood count, and they found the reason for my recent symptoms: a blood sugar of over five hundred! So now, endocrinologists, dietitians, diabetes educators, blood sugar checks, and insulin shots joined the cancer team. My doctors didn't know whether diabetes was a temporary side effect caused by the prednisone, or if I was destined to get diabetes anyway and the leukemia "brought it out early." I rang in 1990 in the hospital not knowing whether my diabetes was a brief setback or a permanent resident. Well, it was here to stay. I am living with and managing my diabetes today. At first, I didn't think having diabetes was a big deal compared to going through cancer, but a lot can go wrong if you don't manage it. What a nasty little gift cancer gave me.

Over the next several weeks, I was admitted to the hospital for blood transfusions, had my radiation treatment, and witnessed my hair fall out and my muscles atrophy. Before ALL, I was able to touch the rim of a basketball hoop. Within a few weeks of lying in bed sick, I wasn't even able to jump high enough to touch the top of a door frame.

Sometime in March, I was admitted to the hospital again because I was experiencing excruciating abdominal pain and I couldn't keep any food or liquids down. The pain kept me in a fetal position, crawling around the floor of my house. My body took another hit with a pancreatitis diagnosis. The cause: l-asparaginase. So, first cancer, then diabetes, and now pancreatitis. This time, I was in the hospital for two weeks. Luckily, no surgery was involved. But doctors believed not eating or drinking anything for a whole month would allow the swelling in my pancreas to go down. So I was sent home with a month's supply of intravenous nutrition— hyperalimentation ("steak & potatoes") and lipids ("whole milk"). While my body was getting supplied with essential nutrients and fats, I experienced hunger pains. At times, I would sneak a small bite of bread, but it always came right back up. "Not yet," my body was telling me.

Something else came home with me too: Demerol. I got dependent on Demerol during my hospital stay and asked for it even when I wasn't in any pain. The first time I had Demerol in the hospital produced an incredible euphoria. I was like, *Wow. This is really, really good stuff.* I asked for it every time that I could, as soon as I could, whether or not I had pain. Fortunately, when I got home, my home nurse decreased the dosage each time he gave it me to the point where I wasn't asking for it anymore.

My last extended hospital stay during my cancer treatment was courtesy of methotrexate. It caused severe sores on my arms, in my mouth, and down my throat. I stayed in the hospital for a week and left with an array of mouth washes and prescriptive solutions to heal the sores.

I heard about Camp Sunshine not long after my diagnosis. Sometime in late winter of 1990, my clinic nurses, Patty Miller and Bonnie Minter, encouraged me to attend. They were key in my recovery and eventually getting me to camp. One day, while I waited my turn to receive treatment, Patty sat me down in a conference room and started a VHS tape. The Beatles' "Here Comes the Sun" blasted through the TV. Next, I saw images of pale, bald-headed kids swimming, playing, laughing, dancing, and singing. There were kids with one leg doing those things. I was angry. I felt robbed. My hair and athleticism were gone; I looked like a ghost; I couldn't eat my favorite foods without vomiting; and I could no longer run without tripping over myself and getting winded. I had lost so much weight that my mom was able to carry me up the stairs, and no mom should be able to carry her fourteen-year-old. I was a mess, and it was a struggle to feel cheerful when I felt miserable and defeated. And I didn't want to go somewhere looking like crap. I wanted to be able to put my best foot forward. So, watching that video, I thought to myself, *That's not me.* I didn't attend camp that year.

My first experience with Camp Sunshine was in the summer of 1991. I wasn't as sick, the treatments were a little easier, and I had hair. But I still didn't feel like having fun. I was miserable. Heck, all the negative energy I was throwing out there was probably the reason my brothers felt they couldn't approach me.

I was a little on edge that first time at camp. I was already a shy kid to begin with, and meeting new people was not my strong suit. Throw in cancer and my shyness only increased. I was amazed, though, at how quickly my inhibition disappeared. Kids were friendly on the bus trip to camp. Some were bald and pale like in the video, but others looked like normal, healthy kids. Some asked me what type of cancer I had. When I arrived at camp, I couldn't believe all of the activities I could do. It was a little too good to be true. Both the adults and campers were welcoming and warm. Nurse Coleen sang a little catchphrase for me every time she gave me my brown envelope of meds during mealtimes. My cabinmates were eager to "show me the ropes" and tell me the "what's what" and "who's who" at Camp Sunshine. Even though they had been there for years and had formed their own groups, they always included me. It was an odd feeling for me to feel so welcomed in a place where I didn't know anyone.

Emil, Matt, Rico, Billy, Brent, Derek, Andy, Joe, Danny—I am not so good with names, but those are engraved in my mind as being part of my fondest memories of camp. I could tell by the way we dressed and spoke that we all came from different backgrounds and had varying personalities. But that didn't matter— we all treated everyone the same. We stayed together.

That first year, we all left the camp dance early to go back to the cabin and play Clue. We would stay up past lights out and talk about life in general, our own cancer battles, and lasting impacts. Who would have thought that teenage boys would want to "just talk"? I guess having cancer has a way of maturing a young person's mind really fast. It's amazing that Camp Sunshine provided an environment where we could live together and become brothers under a rustic cabin roof. Thanks to cancer, we were able to attend Camp Sunshine. Thanks to Camp Sunshine, we became brothers.

Right now, at camp, one of the things that is encouraged with the counselors is having cabin chats.

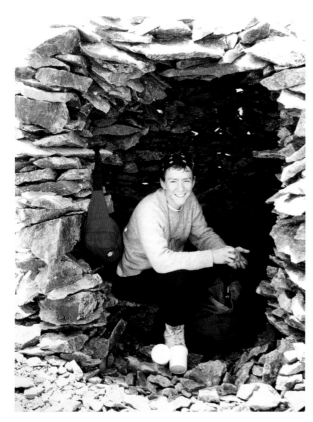

Javi on Camp Sunshine Colorado trip

Well, we were already having them. As a camper that first year, the cabin chats were neat, therapeutic times. We would talk about all kinds of stuff. We would talk about our cancer. We would talk about girls—not crudely or anything, but like, "Wow, it's amazing what she's been through and look at how pretty she is." We respected each other. Sometimes there would be a sobering moment, and it would be up to someone to say, "OK. Enough of this serious stuff, let's laugh!" Then we would cut up and try to make it a little bit lighthearted. Our counselor didn't have to do anything to facilitate that. It was spontaneous.

We would always challenge each other. We never thought, *because we have cancer, we're limited*. We just treated each other as if we didn't have cancer.

It is just amazing the relationships that develop, not only among volunteers but also between volunteers and former campers. I never thought I would be friends with any of the counselors, but I became close to Jeff, who taught the ropes course. Those friendships are something special. They are an everlasting connection. I think it would be hard for any volunteer to forget being there for the roughest part of these kids' lives. The counselors help them get a little bit better.

I never believed that I was going to be in it for the long haul, but my relationship with camp has grown

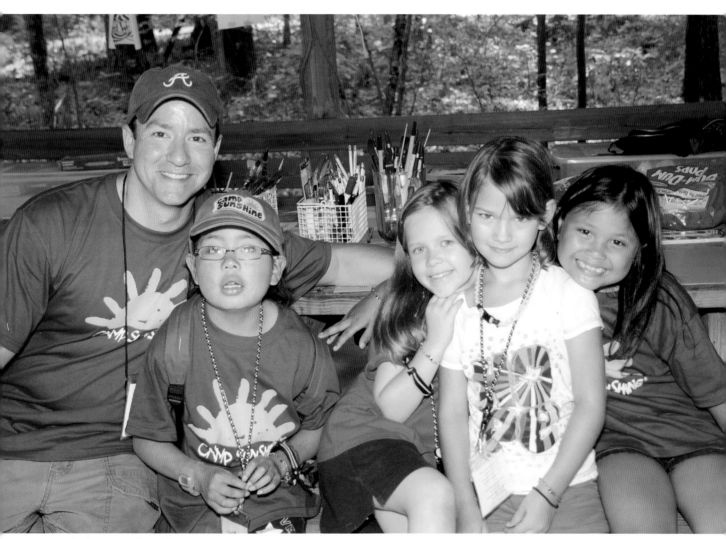

Javi as counselor with campers

from having all the fun a kid could have as a camper to volunteering in a number of capacities as an adult. I went from being a counselor in training (CIT) to a junior week cabin counselor for nine years to the coordinator of the new CIT program, called leaders in training. I help out with the weekend programs (family camps, sibling camps, teen retreats) and am now transitioning onto the Camp Sunshine Advisory Committee after serving on the Board of Directors for five years.

It is hard to believe that the kid who got diagnosed with ALL in 1989 would grow up to serve Camp Sunshine for so many years. It has been a rewarding experience to work alongside the Camp Sunshine staff and volunteers, many of whom were counselors when I was a camper. They're STILL volunteering today! What does that tell you? Humans have such a short attention span that we move on and do other things. We transition into different roles, either becoming parents or grandparents or building careers or moving away. Sometimes life throws things our way, and it is not as easy to do things like Camp Sunshine. So it is quite an accomplishment that throughout camp's thirty-five-year existence, the teamwork and passion to lift these kids' spirits while they battle cancer has endured.

I have been married to my wife, Lisa, for eighteen years. She, too, is a Camp Sunshine volunteer. We have

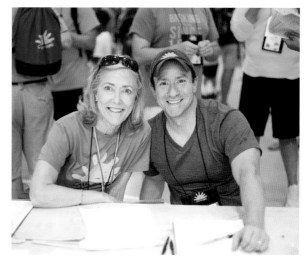

Javi with Sally

a sixteen-year-old daughter, Claudia, and a thirteen-year-old son, Logan. MaPa are living out their retirement years enjoying their six grandkids. My brothers, Luis and Rob, are both married, and each have two kids of their own. All of my family live in Georgia, and we get together frequently. I work as a litigation paralegal, but I would love to find a career where I can coach baseball and work with kids in building up their mental and physical toughness. I want the opportunity to pass along the Camp Sunshine ideals bequeathed to me as a camper.

My nurse, Patty Miller, was key in helping my parents be calm throughout the whole process. Everything was foreign to them. They had no idea what was going to happen. She empathized with them, and somehow, she was able to keep them sane. She encouraged them to keep me eating and drinking and that it would get better. Bonnie Minter was there too. Together, they comforted my parents and offered them advice and guidance when they felt completely helpless and believed I was going to die. They constantly reminded me to not give up, so whenever I was around them, I felt some peace. Patty and Bonnie always made themselves available on the phone if my parents had any questions. Patty and Bonnie became part of the family.

Some people don't come back to camp because they have passed on. There is no guarantee that some of these kids will be around next summer. Joe Brooks, one of my cabin friends, is no longer with us. He died right around the time I was in college. But during that one week at Camp Sunshine, kids live the best they can and don't limit themselves.

What gives Camp Sunshine its legacy is its healing quality. Cancer is tough, and the medicine we take to get better often makes us even sicker. When cancer hits, it breaks kids, and it breaks their families. When a person's spirit and body is broken, there has to be a healing. Over the years, the doctors and nurses at Scottish Rite and Egleston have done wonders to cure these kids physically. Treatment leaves a lot of uncertainty, but there's a place where special people with cancer can fish, sing, dance, and ride horses, Camp Sunshine, where these kids can laugh, smile, and have the most fun they can have. Camp encourages these kids: "You can ride horseback even if you have never seen a horse in your life. You love to sing and dance? Then let's hear it and see it! You can climb this thirty-foot rock wall even if you have one leg. In one day, you can learn to swim! You like art? Well, here's all the arts and crafts you can do! The choice is yours."

Camp Sunshine's influence goes well beyond making an impact during that one week. Over the years, many of these former campers have returned as volunteers to contribute their talents and the same encouragement they received as campers. I have come to realize that Camp Sunshine creates ambassadors who champion the values of hope, strength, patience, and relentlessness. I learned these virtues as a camper, and I hope to pass them along to anyone going through cancer. My spiritual healing would not have been possible without the volunteers who cared.

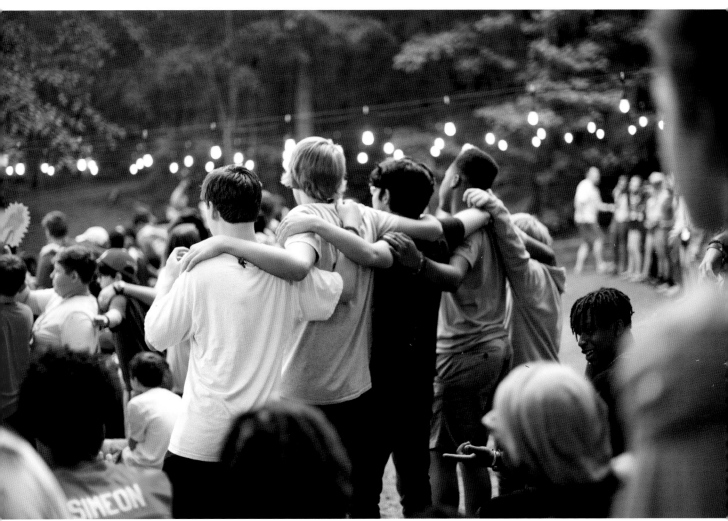

Teen camp boys

Camp Sunshine has a way of "recharging my batteries." I have walked away from every Camp Sunshine program with a renewed feeling that I can face whatever the world throws at me. At Camp Sunshine, I am focused on that day and what I can do to help enrich the lives of kids going through cancer. From the moment campers start arriving, we are geared up and psyched for the week. We make sure that they have the best time they can because it is the one week out of the year when they can experience what they do.

I don't know if I would be who I am today if it weren't for cancer and Camp Sunshine. Cancer or not, this world can be ugly. Maintaining a connection with Camp Sunshine makes everything petty. It is good to know that there is a place where there are good people who make an impact in these kids' lives.

If camp weren't there, all of these teenagers and little kids would just go to clinic and go home and face whatever the world has to give them, without feeling renewed. If that rock wall weren't there, someone who has lost their leg isn't going to experience the rehabilitation that camp offers. Camp says to them, "Who cares if you've got one leg? You can still climb this wall." Well, they will carry that message with them for the rest of their lives.

Camp reminds me that, even as an adult, there's nothing I can't do. Sometimes I can be my own worst enemy. I know this sounds corny, but camp reminds me "you can do anything."

What I want to say to every newly diagnosed child is that there is a place for them, and *this magical place is called Camp Sunshine, and we can't wait to meet you.*

PATTY

Javi is one of my favorite people. He is an amazing young man who has risen above so much, yet he is incredibly humble. Javi is smart, dedicated, full of life, and I am so proud of him. He has fought hard to survive, and I am grateful he survived and is alive today.

I first visited Camp Sunshine in 1986 or 1987, when it was located at Camp Barney Medintz. One of my earliest memories of camp is of Javi running up to me in the amphitheater and giving me a Camp Sunshine friendship bracelet. I have never forgotten that moment because I felt welcomed right away. Whenever I saw Javi at camp, he was always so joyful and happy to see me, which made me feel welcomed and a part of the Camp Sunshine community.

The first year that I visited Camp Sunshine I had been hired as an infusion nurse at Scottish Rite Children's Hospital in Atlanta (now CHOA). I mixed chemotherapy for my first job there, and Javi was one of my patients at the time.

My first time volunteering at Camp Sunshine came a few years later, when Camp Twin Lakes opened in 1993. I was nervous and wondering, *How are they doing chemo at camp?* I remember Bonnie, another camp nurse, administering doxorubicin (chemotherapy); I can still picture her giving chemo in the tiny camp infirmary. I saw that everything was OK; everybody was safe. The kids were truly happy there. I realized, *How cool it was that in this rugged, rural, wonderful place, these kids can get their chemo and continue on with camp activities!*

Mealtimes have always been the heartbeat of camp because that is where everybody is together. I love going to the dining hall and sitting near the amazing counselors. By day two or three of camp, the counselors have all of the campers singing and dancing. The campers are engaged because of how welcomed and connected the counselors make them feel.

I learned a lot with Javi, when I was still fairly new to my oncology nurse role. I loved taking care of him

and his family. He had a couple of younger brothers, and I realized how hard it is for teenagers to go through treatment and how much siblings are impacted by a cancer diagnosis. Even after they go into remission, it seems like the kids with leukemia are in treatment for a long time, and it was powerful to watch Javi during that time blossom from a quiet, scared teenager to a confident and healthy young man.

Javi had to go on insulin because of the steroids we gave him. I knew that diabetes was a potential side effect of steroid treatment, but typically the insulin resistance goes away. This was not the case for Javi. I felt bad; actually, I felt terrible thinking, *my goodness, our treatment does this.* Did it upset him? No. I think Javi, like other Camp Sunshine campers, just learned to live with it. They are so very resilient.

Years later, I visited Javi when he and his wife had their first baby at Northside Hospital. I recall running across the street from my nursing unit at Scottish Rite Children's Hospital to visit him. He wanted me to meet his baby! At the time I didn't fully understand the magnitude of survivorship and fertility; I didn't appreciate the joy of being able to have your own children until I met Javi's baby. I am so grateful for his kids and to have witnessed his joy.

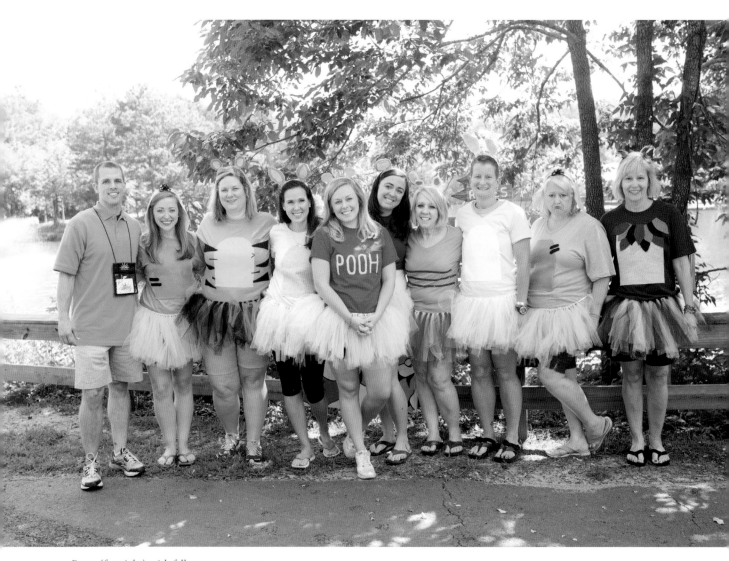

Patty (far right) with fellow camp nurses

I loved taking care of Javi and other Camp Sunshine kids as a new oncology nurse. They kept me in nursing because falling in love with oncology, the patients, and Camp Sunshine sneaks up on you. Oncology nursing grew on me, and my love for it just took over—I was committed!

Camp Sunshine has taught me how precious life is. It has been my privilege to see kids at Camp Sunshine whose parents know they have only months or weeks left. I can't imagine knowing that I had only weeks left with my own child and wanting every minute with them. The fact that those parents share their kids with us during those last months or days or weeks shows how important camp is to them, which amazes me.

I have realized that you cannot know what some of these kids have been through. The effects of their diagnosis and treatment may not be physically obvious but their resilience and courage demonstrates that they have fought the battle. Their experience with cancer, although it may have been years ago, makes them empathetic to what kids in active treatment are going through.

It humbles me how sick some of the kids are. The effort is always to keep kids at camp the whole week, but sometimes, it is not medically an option. If they can't make it through the whole week, that is OK. The counselors make sure the kids do the activities that are most important to them, and the kids enjoy the days they have at camp.

Camp Sunshine has enriched my life tremendously. The true gift for us, as nurses and doctors, is to see how camp changes these kids. I wish that the counselors who have inspired that positive change in the kids all week at camp could see those remarkable changes in the months after camp. It is such a gift for the nurses and doctors to see how camp truly impacts these kids throughout the entire year. We see them standing and sitting up straighter with renewed confidence. We see their continued growth and the connections they form. We see how they want to go back to camp. Camp Sunshine helps these kids become more successful in the world and realize how very special they are. What a gift!

13 It's that connection

Stephanie (Steph) Phillips (August 12, 1986–February 8, 2005; hometown: Fayetteville, Georgia), as told by Paige Phillips Smith, and Christie Powell

PAIGE

When my sister Stephanie was diagnosed with cancer, we had no idea how life changing this experience would be, not just for her but for me. Stephanie grew so much through her summers at Camp Sunshine, gradually moving from a shy camper to a spokesperson for Camp Sunshine, recruiting new kids at the hospital. Even I, as a sibling, found a future path by participating in camp's sibling events. Our parents received so much from camp's outreach.

Steph went to Camp Sunshine for six summers, throughout her treatment. I could see the difference that Camp Sunshine made for Steph. When she first started treatment, she was very much an introvert and was shy about what she was experiencing. Camp was like a complete 180 for her. She arrived with a wig and

went home bald. She did not want to deal with the wig anymore, and she was relieved to be comfortable enough to go out and about without it. She ended up going to prom with just glitter on her head. Winning prom queen that year at camp was amazing for her.

Steph went to camp and realized that there were other kids with cancer and made the best friends of her life there. I remember there was a softball game one summer at camp. Growing up, we all played softball, and Steph played outfield a lot. Steph was in a wheelchair then. She still wanted to play softball, so her friends automatically said, "You're going to play, and we're going to push you around in this wheelchair." She was still able to participate. The friendships she made at camp lasted all year; we had slumber parties at our house all the time for her camp friends. They tried to get together as much as they could; even after Steph died, they came around, and to this day, my family still connects with her friends.

Steph was a quiet person, but she valued camp because of the connections she had with people and the friends she made who understood what her life was like. It's hard for "outsiders" to understand the experience of going through cancer. Her friends in seventh period math class had no idea why she was pale, why she was always in the nurse's office because she was sick. They didn't get it. It is really, really hard to get. At camp, it is a relief not having to explain why someone is bald and has an amputation and a port scar. The kids are who they are, and people at Camp Sunshine accept them for that and understand it.

Besides not being understood, kids with cancer lose a lot of friends when they are diagnosed because their friends don't know how to handle it. They want to be a friend, but they are scared. Their friends are scared that they are going to lose a friend, so they distance themselves a bit to make it easier. That was the hardest part for Steph. Our softball teams were still a good close niche, but we weren't ever as close as we were before she got diagnosed, and very few of her friends from school stuck with her throughout her diagnosis. Then Steph went to camp and gained a whole new group of friends.

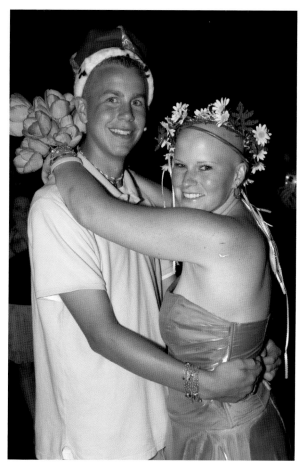

Stephanie at teen camp dance

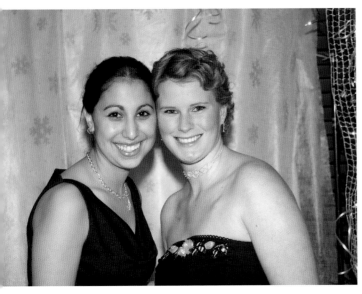
Stephanie (right) with fellow camper at teen camp

Steph also became a spokesperson in the children's hospital for Camp Sunshine. She would go into newly diagnosed patients' rooms and tell them about this wonderful camp and encourage them to go. She would tell them, "It's OK to be a little scared. Soon you'll be comfortable in your own skin." She would explain that camp would normalize them. They would not be an outcast. They would be able to do things that they had been told they couldn't do. They could have

independence, and they would develop the confidence to go out and try something new. Steph told them, "Camp Sunshine is special because it doesn't matter what clique you're in at school, everybody is one clique at camp. The high school jock and the nerd become best friends at camp."

After hearing these messages from Stephanie, I thought, *This is awesome. I'm going to go spend my summers there.* The first time I went to Camp Sunshine for a sibling event, I was in eighth grade. Steph was diagnosed in 2000, when she was in seventh grade. Although I thought I was too cool to go to camp, when I went for sibling weekend, I realized that this was an awesome place. I had a great time. I met Cathy, who volunteers at camp now and is a nurse. We automatically connected, and we remain friends to this day. I was able to make connections on a deeper level with a lot of people. As much as parents try to not single out the child that has cancer, it happens because that kid needs more attention. It was easy for the siblings at camp to relate to each other because it was happening to all of us, that our parents focused on our sister or brother with cancer. To have that sibling weekend to shine was very special. We did a session with a child life worker, and we had to pick out beads that reminded us of our sibling with cancer. I still have the keychain

I made, and I remember what each bead meant to me at that time.

I decided that I wanted to spend my summers volunteering at camp. I wanted to witness how it affected all the other campers like it had my sister. I wanted to help campers achieve their goals and become more comfortable in their own skin, no matter what they were dealt.

I spent ten years on the Camp Twin Lakes staff, including completing their presidential fellowship program. After the fellowship ended in 2009, I became the Camp Twin Lakes program coordinator then camp manager. So, I've been full circle, going to camp as the sibling of a child with cancer to now managing the camp facility. Having a deeper passion and understanding keeps me closer to the mission of Camp Sunshine too.

Looking back, I remember I was in school when Steph first got sick and my mom figured out what was going on with her. I remember that day like it was yesterday. The principal called me up to the front office at school. Mom was there and told me that Steph had a tumor in her hip. She had Ewing's sarcoma.

At that age, I was still unsure of a lot. I didn't understand it. I was in eighth grade, so I obviously knew that having cancer was not good, but I thought Steph

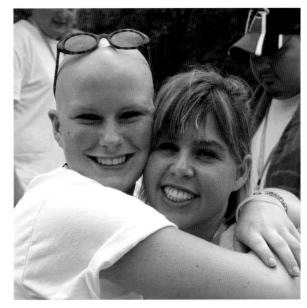

Stephanie with camp counselor

would do chemo and radiation and be fine. For a while, she was. She went into remission for two years but then relapsed. The cancer was in her femur that time. She had her leg and three-fourths of her left hip replaced and then had to go through another round of treatment. She never quite went into remission again. The cancer returned, now in her back and her lungs, and at that point, there was not much else that they could do. Steph had turned eighteen and decided that her body was tired. My mom said it was the hardest decision of her life, but that's what Steph wanted.

Steph died in February 2005. I worked summers at Camp Twin Lakes, and my family did the Remember the Sunshine (bereavement camp) in the fall of 2005. That was the first one that we did, and it was the hardest because it was the year Steph died. Some of her cabinmates were working at Camp Twin Lakes and were present at the program. It was really hard for my family. They were thinking, *Steph should be here with you guys doing this.*

My mom is super strong and was able to deal with Steph's passing over time, so sometimes it seems funny to us that we still visit the Camp Sunshine House and go back for every Remember the Sunshine weekend we can. But for the parents who are new—who have just lost their child—those bereavement weekends give them hope that they can make it through this. My parents have been living for more than ten years without their daughter, and they know that life does go on. They also remember the connections they made through family weekends, and the support they received from other parents who were in the same boat. So they step in and become mentors for the new ones.

Steph and I were sixteen months apart. I have an older sister, Shannon, who is four years older than me. I think I dealt with it a lot better than Shannon, because the Remember the Sunshine weekends are still hard for her. It's still very healthy and helpful for her to go; we just grieve differently.

What happens at camp has such a ripple effect on the families and those around them. Once the families can understand it and begin to network, it's easier for them to cope, which then ripples out to their friends and work environment. It's that connection piece that comes up again and again.

Christie Powell was one of Steph's main nurses at camp and in the hospital. She meant the world to my family and still does. She is amazing and great at what she does. She'll give the tough love when necessary. That's what our family thrives on because that's what we've all always grown up with. She can connect and meet her patient wherever their need is; if they need tough love, she can give it to them. If they need more of just love and attention, she can give them that—whatever they need.

Being with Steph at camp enhanced their relationship as patient and nurse when they returned to the hospital. There is something special about seeing your nurses and doctors at camp, not giving you shots, but playing and having fun and being people too. They aren't trying to hurt you, often the image kids get when

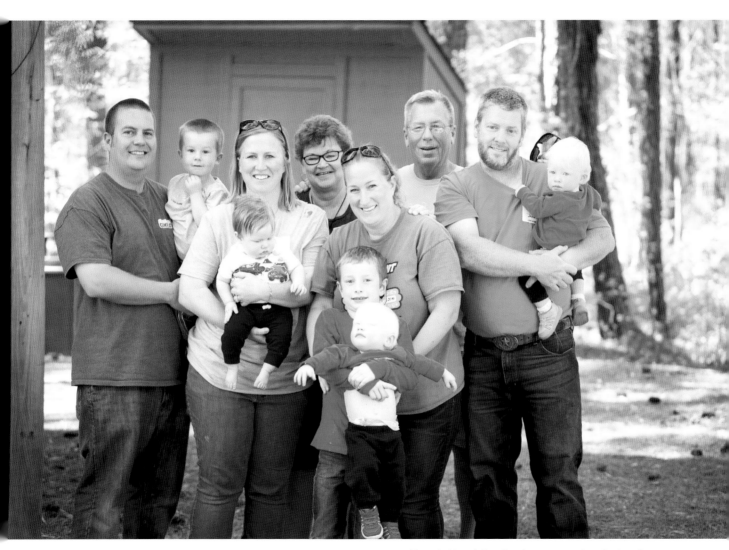

Paige (front left) with her family at Remember the Sunshine

they go to the doctor or hospital. When the nurses and doctors are able to go to camp, they can be humanized, and the kids realize that they're doing it for the good. So once Steph got comfortable, she was not afraid to go up to Christie and ask her to do things, like join her at the pool. I could see Steph doing that but only at Camp Sunshine. Steph was very fierce but shy. She would not do that anywhere else.

Camp Sunshine is where we have the strongest kids in Georgia. They're able to thrive and persevere through whatever challenges in order to go to camp. The fact that campers on hospice care can go, and their families are OK with that even though they don't know what the week holds is a huge message of support. Where else would that happen? A few years ago, I saw a sister drop off a camper who was on hospice. The sister was leaving with a smile, and I was thinking, *How in the world could she be leaving with a smile?* I stopped and greeted her, and she said she was so thrilled that her sister could spend one more week at camp. She knew that this is where her sister wanted to be no matter what happened. I wondered if I would have been that strong if I were in her shoes.

CHRISTIE

I knew I wanted to be a pediatric oncology nurse in high school. I had read a book called *Children's Hospital*, which, I believe, was written about Children's Hospital of Philadelphia. Each chapter was about a different patient or a different family or a nurse that worked there. The patients had cancer, cystic fibrosis, and other chronic illnesses. I just loved that book, and I knew that that was what I wanted to do.

When I first graduated from nursing school, Tricia Benson interviewed me for a job on the oncology unit at Egleston Children's Hospital (now Children's Healthcare of Atlanta). She was the unit director at the Aflac Cancer Center. Within the first five minutes of my interview, I heard about this awesome place called Camp Sunshine. Tricia was saying, "You can have this job, but the best thing about it is going to this place called Camp Sunshine. You have to go." That was my first introduction to camp, and I *had* to become a part of it. It wasn't even an option.

When Tricia asked me to go to camp, I said, "Yes, that sounds great!" I had no hesitations. That was partly due to the way Tricia delivered the message. She said, "You'll be doing this because I know you're going to love it. I know it's going to suit your personality and you'll be awesome at it. Camp's amazing, and in one year, we'll have you there." I had just missed Camp Sunshine that summer, so I had to wait a full year. I went the following summer, in 1994, and I just fell in love.

My first year at camp, I was on the activity staff doing horseback riding. Usually, no one ever wants to do that because it's hot, people aren't familiar with horses, and everyone's uncomfortable. I grew up with horses, so it was a great experience for me. I was comfortable out there. I think one of the coolest things about horseback riding was that a lot of magic happens. Most of these kids that go to Camp Sunshine have not had exposure to horses or been on horses before. What they witness up there on the horse is amazing, whether it is their first time riding, or they have had their leg or arm amputated and didn't think they could ever get on a horse again, or they are blind from a brain tumor and didn't think getting on a horse would ever be possible for them. It was a gift for me to do horseback riding my first year because it was a neat lead-in to camp. It exposed me to what Camp Sunshine was like and the magic that occurs there.

At the hospital, as soon as we get kids with a new diagnosis, we tell them, "This is a horrible deal. We're sorry that you're here, but there are a lot of cool things that we're going to share with you and that you'll be able to participate in because of cancer." Of course, Camp Sunshine is the main thing, so we start talking to them about that right away.

Camp Sunshine has changed a lot over the years. It has tripled in size, as far as programs, activities, and the accommodations. So much thought has been put into this place, and we are truly lucky to have a facility like Camp Twin Lakes. Now we have programming and support year-round for kids and their families. These programs are a good way to get kids involved because it is easier for families to jump in or engage in activities like family camp or a teen weekend before they are willing to commit to a week of summer camp.

I think of the connections at Camp Sunshine on a couple of different levels. I think it is amazing to see patients and families in this atmosphere, in this part of their life, and not just in the clinic. I think campers and families also see us medical providers in a different light when we are at camp with them. We are not just their nurses or doctors; we are regular people like they are. It is cool for me to see them engage with their friends and participate in regular activities.

What I love is when a camper's light begins to shine again. It gets dimmed and dulled by chemo, radiation, and all the treatments they get because they feel so poorly. It is impossible for cancer not to take a toll on them. Going to Camp Sunshine lights their spark again. The campers do not believe it is going to happen, even resist going. They might fight you tooth and nail about it! No one can understand what camp looks or feels like until they have been there and experienced it. That is true for the nurses and the staff, as well as the campers.

That feeling of connectedness we all share is powerful: with fellow volunteers, whether it is the nurses or cabin counselors. We are all there with the same mission, and it is satisfying to share that goal. It's heartwarming to see all of us from the Aflac Cancer Center joking around and laughing, watching the kids do the zip line and the pamper pole, and being able to go back to the hospital and share those experiences and stories with the other staff who cannot make it to camp. It is very meaningful, and it fills our cup. Going to camp rejuvenates me so I can go back to the hospital and keep doing what I am doing, day in and day out.

I think of camp as extended family, really. These are the people I have known, most of them for a very, very long time, through thick and thin and through all of life's ups and downs. We all continue to make this work, to be a part of it, to share, and to laugh and cry together. I feel that way about the staff I work with at the Aflac Cancer Center, as well. Camp is just an extension of that community in a lot of ways. The volunteers are like family.

There are so many life lessons to be gained at camp. I think the biggest takeaway is that life is hard. Life can throw us a lot of curveballs, but how we approach and handle them is how we're going to have an outcome. If we take those curveballs and hard times and make something positive out of them, then we're moving in a forward direction. That's what I see at camp all day long. I see these kids persevering. They're resilient. They go out there after surgeries and amputations, and they're doing the climbing wall. They're making friends. They're laughing again.

I think to myself, *No problem that I have is so significant that I can't overcome it.* Camp puts everything into perspective. It just makes me realize that every day is a gift. Yes, I'm going to have troubles along the way, but I have people around me who support me and love me and care about me. That is what we hope the campers leave with, and we feel that way too. You can't be at Camp Sunshine and not feel that.

Steph was an amazing, amazing girl. I was just totally blown away by her. She was one of my patients when I first became a nurse practitioner, and she had a tough journey. When her cancer came back, she continued to fight it; her inner strength and peace never wavered.

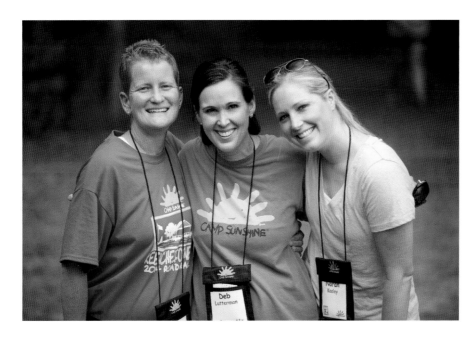

*Christie (left) with
fellow camp nurses*

She always had this very quiet strength and courage about her. She handled every step of the way, throughout her journey, with this amazing grace. When I think of her, I think of laughter, warmth, and grace.

I remember Steph at camp. She immediately fit right in. The girl had no fear. She had a quiet confidence. She was a great athlete. She was so warm and personable that she befriended everybody right away. Everybody loved Stephanie. She was one of those people that everyone gravitated toward because her energy was so positive and warm. That is no surprise, if you know her family. Paige is the same way. Her parents are the same way.

Steph loved this place. Camp was heaven to her. I remember a lot of laughter with her at camp. I vividly remember her getting ready for the dance with her cabinmates, memories of them laughing and having fun together with all of their makeup on. I think a lot about Steph's smiling and her joy. That's what I remember

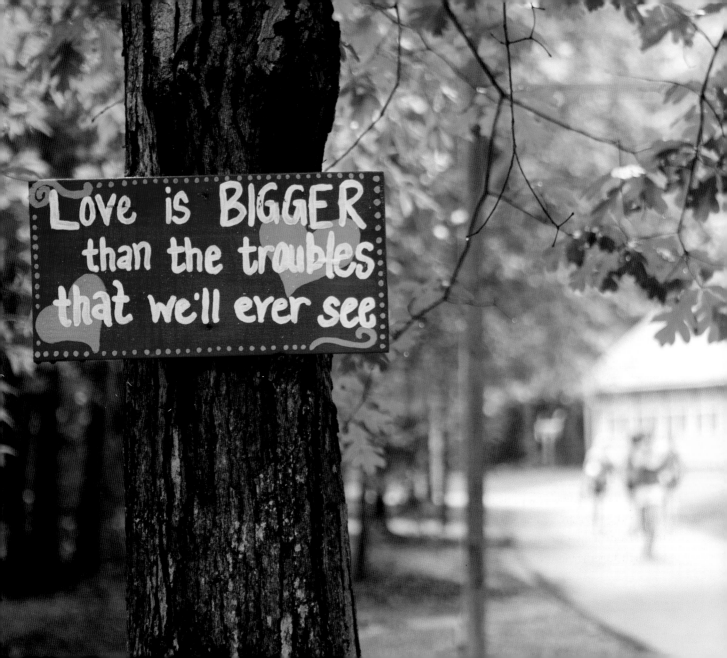

about her being at Camp Sunshine. When I'm at camp, I think about Steph and all the kids who are no longer with us, who loved it. They are here in spirit with us. At the camp remembrance ceremony, I was thinking that the "Stephanies" out there are the campers that have taught us so much. They are the ones who said, "Live every day to your fullest. Love every day. Don't let little things get in your way. Don't get hung up on things that don't matter. Just be present and live every day in the best way you can."

I think about that message when I am at camp and every day, and I feel so thankful that I have that daily reminder in my life. So many people don't. It is so easy to get hung up on the little things, but you don't when you are at camp and when you are around these kids. Stephanie and so many others have taught me that lesson, and I try my hardest to live by it, for them, for myself, for my family, and for everyone that I love.

Camp Sunshine keeps me balanced. It's great for me professionally and personally on so many levels. Professionally, I think it gives me street credit with the kids at work to be out there with them at camp. They know how much they mean to me when they see me at camp. We are so lucky because we take away so much from camp ourselves. It is fun for us to be there, to laugh together and do things together. Personally,

camp teaches me so much about life and living and loving. Camp is a good reminder to take away that lesson and don't forget it. Apply it to your life.

I think what makes Camp Sunshine most special is that these kids get to be kids again. They get to feel normal around their peers. One of our campers said it best: "I was basically telling my cabin that I was nervous and afraid. I wasn't sure I wanted to be here, and they got it. They really got it." That puts camp into words for me because there are not a lot of places for these kids where people "get it." Yes, as their care providers we know what they are going through, but we are not experiencing it. At camp, the kids are surrounded by peers who have experienced it or are still experiencing it. To hear of a kid yelling at her father the whole way because she doesn't want to go, getting dragged out of the car "kicking and screaming," and then within hours, loving it and saying that she never wants to leave? That's Camp Sunshine, right there.

That is one of the best things about this place. That is what we all love, and that's what makes camp magical. It fills camp with love, and the thing is, you cannot put it into words or explain it to somebody until they're there and they experience it. If you go out there and you can't wrap your heart around that, then I don't know why.

14 Camp blocks out all the noise

Will Hennessy (born February 3, 1997; hometown: Marietta, Georgia)
and Kenneth Kretschmar

WILL

It was right before my sixth birthday: January 19, 2003. My left leg had been hurting. I was out playing basketball with my dad, my sister, and my best friend. By the time the game ended, my leg hurt so badly that my dad literally had to carry me into the kitchen and put me on the kitchen table so my mom could have a look at it. The next morning was Saturday, and my mom took me to an urgent care center. After they took an X-ray, the doctor called everyone—all the doctors, all the nurses—into a room to look at it. When they all came back to our room, the doctor told us to go to the children's hospital. I believe he thought it was cancer, was pretty sure it was cancer, but he didn't want to say for sure.

I remember being in the hospital room when they told me I had cancer. I remember looking at the X-ray, and my left leg looked like an eaten-up apple core. Even though I was only six years old, I could tell that image wasn't the way it should be. I could see something was wrong. I still remember my mom specifically asking, "Kids can have cancer?" It blew her mind to think, *my kid has cancer.*

I was diagnosed with Ewing's sarcoma; it's a rare cancer that most often occurs in and around the bones. I was in kindergarten at the time, and one of the parents at my school had had Ewing's sarcoma back in the 1970s. The doctors had talked to my parents about amputating the left leg below the knee, but this parent at our school was so helpful and encouraged us to get a second opinion. We went to MD Anderson in Houston.

I remember the doctor there drawing a picture of my leg on the examining table paper. He showed my parents exactly what he wanted to do to save my leg. He said, "I think we can do this. I think we can save the leg." My parents believed I had so much life ahead of me, so to save the leg—to have it for the rest of my life—was important and a deciding factor.

I was placed in a clinical trial. I underwent eight rounds of chemotherapy before leg surgery and fourteen rounds in all. It was a rough time. I remember the doctors saying that they were going to kill me with chemo. That's how much chemo I was getting. With my chemo, they were basically putting poison into a six-year-old kid's body. But it's the only thing strong enough to kill the cancer. I remember at one point the medical team was flushing out my port (port-a-cath), and they did it too fast, and I puked all over the floor.

Somehow my body was able to go through it all. The tumors were shrinking. You know, having cancer as a child is not something that comes with an instruction book. You know, the doctors don't give you an instruction manual: *Here's How to Have Cancer at Age Six*. I think about my parents, what they were going through at that time, and I think about my sister, Clare, who was eight years old at the time. I don't know how she felt having a younger brother who could die any day. The worry she must have carried!

In July 2003, I had surgery at MD Anderson. Doctors removed ten centimeters of my left fibula and inserted a screw to stabilize my leg. Because the piece of bone that was removed is not weight bearing, they didn't put anything in there to replace the bone. There is nothing there, just a gap in my leg. I couldn't play contact sports to avoid the risk of a compound fracture. But I will take a gap in my leg and no-contact sports over a leg amputation any day.

It is funny what you remember as a kid. What I remember most about my surgery was that my mom and dad had promised me a Chick-fil-A sandwich when it was all over. So, as my mom was waiting at the hospital, my dad was driving all over Houston looking for a Chick-fil-A sandwich. That is the only thing I remember from the actual day of surgery—that sandwich! The next day was the MLB All-Star game in Houston. I watched the All-Star game in my room with my dad and mom. The doctor came into the room, and he was a big baseball fan.

After surgery, I began physical therapy to regain function of my left leg—a wheelchair, then crutches followed. I started first grade on time with my class.

Although contact sports were out of the question, I played other sports and eventually channeled my interest in sports into a sports management degree at the University of Michigan, where I study now. My mom went to the University of Michigan, and I fell in love with the school from going to football games there growing up. The winters are brutal, but my years at Michigan have given me some outstanding opportunities, like being the head student manager of the Wolverines football team. That position has given me a chance to be part of the team. Since I couldn't play football, it's the next best thing for me. I have also worked on the promotions staff during the first season at the Atlanta Braves SunTrust Stadium, overseeing young fans in the Kids' Zone. I took a week off from that job to volunteer for junior week at Camp Sunshine. It just has such a special place in my heart, and I didn't want to miss out.

I have been cancer-free for years. I continue to do all the survivor clinics at Emory University. Because of the chemotherapy, I am at risk of possibly developing heart problems, so I see a cardiologist. It sounds funny, but looking back, I honestly can't imagine my life without cancer and the journey it led me on. I don't wish it on anyone, but cancer got me ready for the rest of my life. I also believe it brought my family even closer

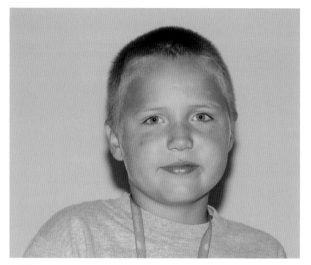

Will, junior camper

together. We were always close, but we are so tight now, and that's a great thing.

I think all of us in my family feel it is important to be huge advocates for fighting cancer and to help other families affected by it. There were families who were there for us, and we want to pay it forward and be there for others. When I was diagnosed, there was a kid at my elementary school who had leukemia. His family members were like angels from God who came down to help us. We want to be those people for other families who are facing this battle. There is no book about how to handle it. The only people who truly know about the experience are the people who have lived through it.

I first heard about Camp Sunshine right after my diagnosis. I learned about family camp from the family of Carter, who was a patient at Egleston. There was so much going on at that time, and I remember my parents saying, *What? You want us to pick up everything and go to a camp in the middle of Georgia and spend an entire weekend there?* But we did, and by Sunday, our family was entirely refreshed and functioning at a whole other level. From that point on, I was hooked on Camp Sunshine.

Carter became my best friend. Believe it or not, we were diagnosed on the same day with the same diagnosis. That summer we attended junior camp together. It was just incredible to be with kids for a whole week, kids who had gone through similar things. For most kids, when they are at school or in their community, they're probably the only kids with cancer. When they walk into Camp Sunshine, nobody cares that they have cancer. It does not matter if they are bald or have an amputation below the knee or have a prosthetic. It is just a community of kids who want to have fun and be together to have a good time.

The first year, my parents were more hesitant than I was about camp. They had typical concerns: *He's out in the middle of nowhere! What if something goes wrong?* But I convinced them. I told them, "I have friends there, and I am at peace when I am with them." As a kid going through cancer, I had to have my parents and the other adults, the doctors and nurses who were constantly taking care of me, around all the time. They had to be there to keep me alive. At camp, I got to be on my own, to be whoever I wanted to be for a while, to just be a kid. As a cancer patient, I was confined to a hospital room and a hospital bed and a very specific routine. But at Camp Sunshine, I suddenly had some of my freedom back. I remember I took advantage of that freedom by doing things like having chocolate milk every single day at every single meal. At home we were allowed to have chocolate milk sometimes because it was more like a treat. But at camp, I could just go for it!

A lot of my earliest and most treasured memories involve my friendship with Carter. We were in Cabin Twenty-One together. Our counselors were great. We used to trade Pokémon cards. My best memory is going frog hunting. We'd sneak down to the lake at night, catch frogs, eat homemade ice cream, and tell ghost stories. Carter couldn't walk at the time, and I remember putting him in a buggy and making sure he didn't miss out on anything.

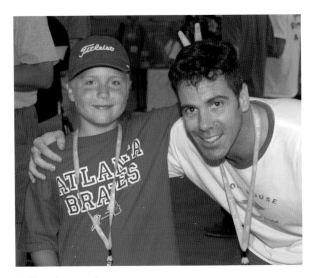

Will with counselor

Carter and I did not get to have a long history of summer camps together. He relapsed and died in 2004. He was seven years old. That is what makes the earliest memories even more special to me. I got to see Carter at his truest self, and I will always be grateful for that. Thinking about Carter and our times together at camp doesn't bring back sad memories; it brings back nothing but great memories. That is the way it is with Camp Sunshine.

It's been twelve years of camp now for me. When I graduated from camp, I became a CIT (counselor in training). I love Camp Sunshine. The impact it has on so many lives, so many populations—not just the campers, but their families, the volunteers, the volunteer nurses, the medical staff—is incredible. So, becoming a CIT was my way to give back.

There is something so special about Camp Sunshine. It is the community, the bonding, and the laughter. There is so much joy. Those are my friends, the friends I have grown up with. I can literally go without seeing them for a whole year, but there is something about camp that when we all get back together, we just pick up right where we left off.

It is a bond like no other. I honestly know that if I ever needed them, I could call ten different people from Camp Sunshine right now, and they would be there for me. We will always be there for each other. There are very few people you meet in your life whom you can say that about. But I know I can count on my camp community, and they know that they can count on me. Like my friend Alex, who was my cabinmate for twelve years. Alex's mother passed away, and I was one of the first people he called. I went to the funeral, and when he saw me, his face lit up. I believe it brought him some

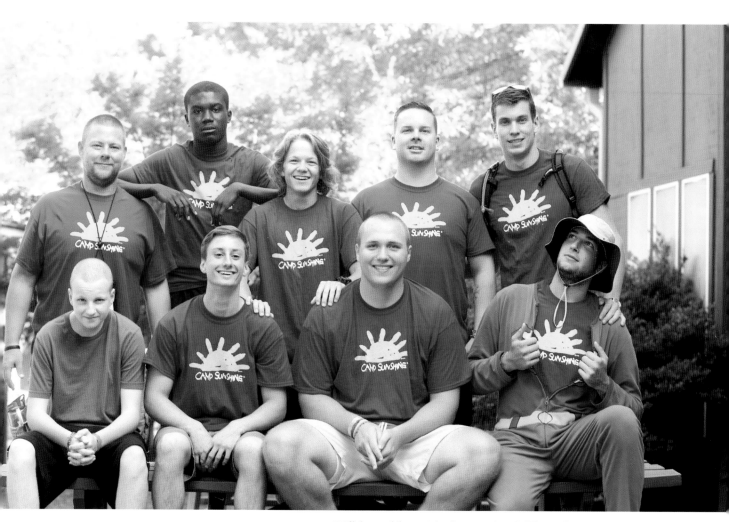

Will (second from right, front row) with fellow cabinmates, teen camp

comfort to know his camp family was there for him and is always there for him.

During my Camp Sunshine years, I really bonded with Kenneth Kretschmar. He is a former camper himself and was my cabin counselor for three years. He had Ewing's sarcoma as a kid, too, and I think having the same kind of cancer helped me identify with him. He was a kind of father figure to me. It wasn't anything specific. It was just his being there for me. I remember having the opportunity to go on Camp Sunshine's outdoor adventure trip to Colorado. Kenneth was going, and I knew it would be awesome. Hiking together and hanging out for a week allowed me to get to know him. Mostly it was just being goofy and kidding around and enjoying each other's company. We stay in touch; we shoot each other a text just to check in and say hi, just to see how each other is doing.

For me, it has been so cool to see the development of individual campers over twelve years. You see kids come in their first year, and maybe they are going through chemo or other treatment, and maybe they are very sick. And then you see those same kids the next year and the next, and maybe one year they are on treatment and the next year they are off. And then to see them maybe four years later, and these kids are well again. There is nothing better than that.

From day one, people are going about one hundred miles per hour at camp. Everybody there wants the same thing: to make the most out of every single minute, every single day. No one wants to be a member of the childhood cancer club, but I can tell you, once you are in, you want to make the most of every moment you've been given. It is an unspoken bond between us all. We all understand why we are there. But while we are there, cancer is not going to stop us. Cancer will never define who we are. We are not going to let it.

I completely understand why kids hesitate about going to camp. I mean, going off without your parents and being in the middle of Georgia for a week with a lot of people that you don't know—that sounds intimidating! But I can also say that ultimately Camp Sunshine changed my life forever. It is a true community, a community of friends who are more like family. No one there focuses on you as a person with cancer; everyone there focuses on you as an individual. Logically, it doesn't make sense that all this can happen to you at a summer camp. But you have to take a leap of faith and see for yourself.

The spirit of Camp Sunshine lives in everyone who goes. We come from different socioeconomic backgrounds, different ethnic backgrounds, different schools, and different walks of life. But at camp, it doesn't matter. It doesn't matter who you were before camp; it matters who you are now, who you truly are. Camp Sunshine blocks out all the noise of the outside world. And being in a place where that kind of spirit rules rarely happens in this world.

KENNETH

I am a childhood cancer survivor. I was diagnosed in 1988 at age nine with Ewing's sarcoma, one week before camp began. I had to start chemo right away, so I couldn't go to camp that year. My first year at Camp Sunshine was in 1989.

I had never been to camp of any sort before and certainly not an overnight camp away from my home and family. This was a whole new experience for me. My parents may have had some fears or concerns about it but not me. Camp was a blast from the start! I remember having to walk long distances on crutches over gravelly roads when I first got there, but there were golf carts too. So I got to ride in a golf cart from place to place a lot of the time, which was its own kind of fun.

The most important thing was I met people that year that are still part of my life today. There were lots of kids with a bunch of counselors in the cabin all at the same time. A closeness developed; those first camp experiences started a whole journey that is still happening now. After the experiences I had as a kid at Camp Sunshine, I can't imagine not giving back.

Times change; things change. But still I try to do the same things for the campers today that my counselors did for me when I was young. Camp is a place to be normal at a time in your life when things are anything but normal. You are *the* kid with cancer. There are not a whole lot of kids who have cancer, not in your school, not in your neighborhood, not in your community. You are *the* one. But you go to Camp Sunshine, and suddenly, you are just a normal kid again because everybody's got cancer.

Camp becomes a part of you. I knew before I graduated that I wanted to go back as a CIT. I had missed two years of camp in high school because I was playing sports. Football was such a love for me, and I had worked so hard to come back from cancer to be able to play again. So I had to make the decision between Camp Sunshine and football for two years. But even with missing that time, I knew I was going to stay involved in camp and become a volunteer counselor myself.

I have been involved with Camp Sunshine for twenty-eight years. My wife, Angie, volunteers too. I

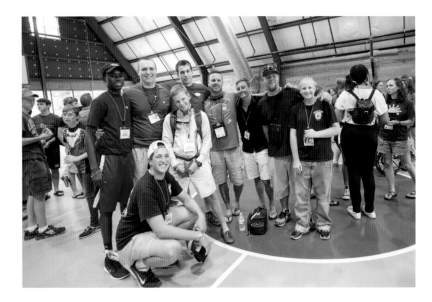

Will (back row, second from left) with fellow campers

roped her into volunteering the first time, but once she got there, she was hooked. We have been working both junior and senior weeks together for twelve years; we also volunteer for several camp programs throughout the year. I go on the Colorado trip, and we also usually volunteer for a family camp, Remember the Sunshine, sibling camp, and teen retreats.

Geographically, Camp Sunshine has changed. We've moved from Camp Barney Medintz, a rugged, rustic site in north Georgia to Camp Twin Lakes in Rutledge.

That ruggedness and sense of adventure added a little something to the overall camp experience. But today we make up for it in other ways with the excellent facilities and all the great programs and opportunities we can offer campers.

The heart of camp hasn't changed and never will. That family feeling, knowing how deeply these people care about each other does not change. No matter who happens to be at camp at any given time in any given year, I know that love is there. These people may have different life experiences than I have had, or they may come from different walks of life, but at camp, we all share the same goals. That does not change.

As I have gotten older, I think the connectedness of Camp Sunshine takes on even more importance. Today technology and social media make it possible to keep up with people even easier, and that is great. Camp has always been about knowing that people were there for you. They are your friends; they are like family. The confidence, the hope, the love, the sharing, and the moral values that are shared and encouraged at camp were instilled in me while I was there as a young kid and are values that I will take with me throughout the rest of my life. There was a shared thinking; I knew that it didn't matter what I was going through because I could get through it with everyone there surrounding and supporting me.

Take someone like Bubbles. I don't remember a time in my life, not one occasion, when I did not get a card from Bubbles. You just always know these people are there for you. I remember Steve Davol would always make it a point to pick me up at home once or twice a year to go to the movies or hang out together. Steve passed away, but to this day, I stay very connected with his sister, Lisa. Even if camp is just that one week out of the year, even if you don't talk to these people for a

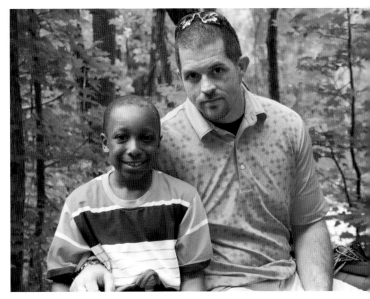

Kenneth with camper

solid year until the next camp rolls around, when you see them, it is like you have not been away for any time at all. The connection happens in an instant, and you just pick up right where you left off.

When my mom passed away this year, about ten people from Camp Sunshine showed up at the funeral and more than one hundred people from camp were in touch to express their condolences and to see how I was doing. Camp is just a unique connection.

I think I bring a lot from my experiences at camp and my fight with cancer to my coaching. I am a high school coach in football, wrestling, and track. I try to create a supportive environment similar to that of Camp Sunshine, where I instill camaraderie among my players. I base my coaching around them as individuals, recognizing each athlete as an individual, while at the same time building the kids up as a team. For me, being a coach is about trying to teach a player not just about being a better athlete but also being a productive young man, a good citizen, and a good person who is going to do the right thing.

These core beliefs were instilled in me by my family, but they were reinforced at Camp Sunshine. I think there's something about hearing these messages from people who are not your direct family. Maybe kids will listen to me because it's *not* coming from their parents. I think that is the way it was for me at camp. Those messages, *you are tough, never quit, don't give up, you can do anything you set your mind to*, you hear them from your parents, but it's also great to hear them from other people who know you and care about you.

I was Will Hennessy's counselor; he was in my cabin for ten-, eleven-, and twelve-year-old boys, so I have known him a long time. Will had Ewing's sarcoma, which is what I had, so we had that diagnosis in common. I had been a sports guy my entire life, and Will was an athlete. He was a big kid, and the cancer had limited him to where he wasn't playing sports when he first came to camp. So we had the same diagnosis and the same love of sports, and I think those two things brought us together from the very beginning. One thing I try to keep in mind and tell the guys I coach, guys like Will, is that all athletes are healthier at some points than at others; everybody has to go through adjustments. So even if Will couldn't play contact sports, I remember playing a lot of dodgeball with him and the boys in my cabin. We played dodgeball down the center of the cabin, and these guys threw a ball at the front door of that cabin with all their might, and just blew that door wide open! That game created a bond between us all that lasts to this day. I text these guys every couple of months to see how they are doing and what they are up to. It's a lifelong bond.

Will is a very driven young man and very compassionate. He is such a big bear of guy and I love to see how compassionate he can be—he has a truly heartfelt caring about anybody and everybody he meets. He is also a very smart guy. Overall, he is just a strong and awesome young man.

Let me tell you a favorite story about Will—it was when we were in Colorado, on a backpacking camp trip. When you get there, they give you a backpack filled with stuff you are going to need. They had to find a double XL for Will so that it would fit him, and it is filled with all kinds of stuff. Will ends up carrying not just his stuff but everybody else's. I was standing beside him before he put his backpack on, and I can tell you that that backpack was so big, it came up to my armpit! I mean, I could fit in it. I was joking with him and said, "I'm getting in it," and I did. And Will stood up and lifted the backpack with me in it!

That trip was a special time for me, as it was for Will. First to have been a cabin counselor for these kids when they are so young and at the very beginning of their cancer journey and then to be with them again when they were older and wrapping up their time at camp was awesome. But it is not just the connection between Will and me or the other guys and me. It is awesome to see how the bond and connection between the guys themselves continues to grow too. These guys are a whole lot bigger now and much more mature than when I first met them. But that bond between them? It is not much different now from when they were first together. It is just stronger.

As crazy as it sounds, I *wouldn't want not to have had cancer* because of this life, these connections, and these people I have in my life today. As bad as the disease is, the entire experience has made me who I am today, and Camp Sunshine is a big part of that. Camp is about love and understanding. The people, especially the counselors who've had cancer themselves, give you complete understanding and a whole lot of love. And those who have not had cancer may not be able to give you complete understanding, but they give you the love.

It is empathy, not sympathy, that you find at Camp Sunshine. At camp, it's like *OK, we empathize with you. Now this is where we can go from here, if you're willing to join us.* At camp, you can share as much or as little as you want about your cancer journey. You can talk about it if you want to and not talk about it if you don't want to. Don't get me wrong; there is a lot of talking that happens at camp. Amazingly, the bond that happens in those moments of sharing is different from anything else I have ever experienced, and it is an unbreakable bond.

Like so many of the volunteers, I could easily have chosen different things to do with my summers, but I choose Camp Sunshine. I will always go back. Life situations might keep me away one year or another, but I will always go back. There are people at camp who just get it. They go one year, then they go back again, and then they stay for life. They cannot imagine not going to Camp Sunshine. I'm so grateful to be with them.

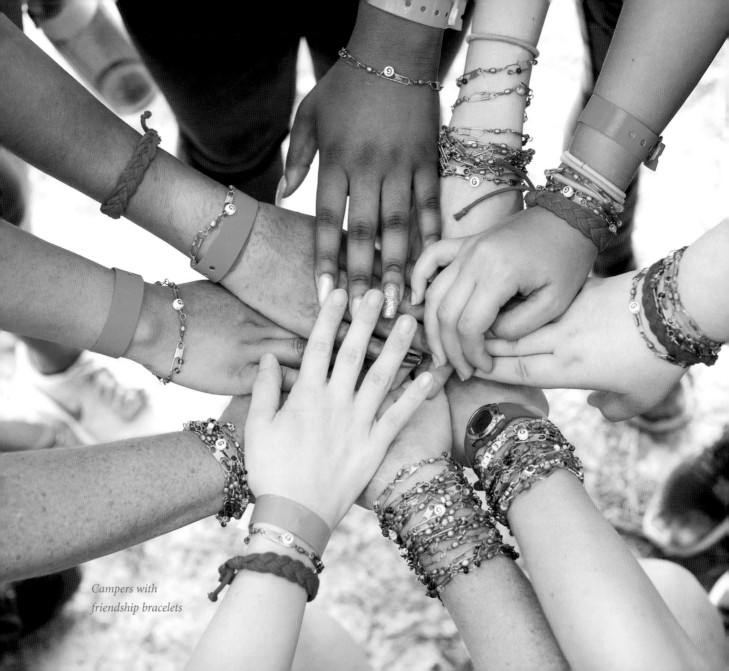

*Campers with
friendship bracelets*

Epilogue

Every year since our first camp session in 1983, each Camp Sunshine camper and volunteer is given a bracelet: a simple circle of fishing swivels and colored beads. You can find these bracelets, which are meant to symbolize the bonds of friendships forged at camp, in the pictures featured throughout this book—from a single chain dangling off the wrist of a new camper, to decades worth of bracelets covering counselors' forearms or strung into long, elaborate necklaces. Some campers and volunteers, like my late husband Hamilton, never take these bracelets off, proudly displaying their connection to Camp Sunshine year-round.

These bracelets are a fitting symbol of the connectedness of the Camp Sunshine community. The connections made at camp are like a thread that stitches each one of us together—a bond that is immeasurable and immutable—drawn stronger by our shared experiences with cancer. This thread empowers everyone in the Camp Sunshine community to carry the powerful love, unending support, and deep sense of belonging that camp has given them throughout their lives.

The power of this connection and community was palpable that first year at Camp Sunshine; I always knew we would be taking camp home with us. But what I could have never known is how cancer would be woven through my life. Two years after starting camp, my husband, Hamilton, was diagnosed with his first cancer—a non-Hodgkin's lymphoma. We found ourselves on the other end of the support structure we had hoped to build as we began to hear from our Camp Sunshine family. Treatment at National Cancer Institute necessitated a move to Bethesda, Maryland, with our nineteen-month-old son, Hamilton Jr. Soon

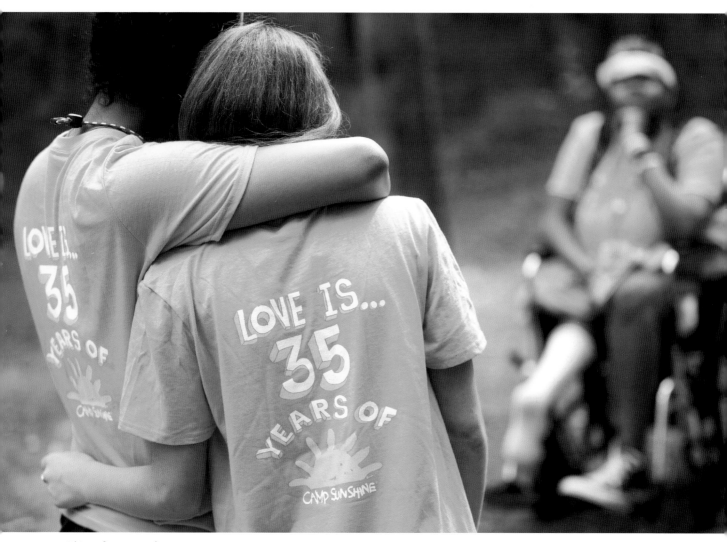

Thirty-five years of camp

after arriving, we received a very large box containing a scrapbook of cards, drawings, and notes from all of the Camp Sunshine campers and volunteers offering Hamilton hope, encouragement, and advice.

This early diagnosis and treatment were just the beginning. Hamilton had several more diagnoses over our twenty-seven years of marriage until his death in May 2008 from malignant mesothelioma. Throughout those years, he was buoyed by his deep connection to the Camp Sunshine community. Hamilton drew from camp's support and continued to find ways to make a difference in people's lives, establish connections, and advocate for all cancer patients and the oncology community.

Witnessing the decades of connections made at Camp Sunshine—and the power that a single moment with others can have—reinforces my belief that we can all make a difference. We can make things better in our everyday lives and in our communities by being aware of gaps and needs. The most powerful thing we can do is to simply be present in any given moment, making a connection with another human being.

In 1982, when I was planning our first summer camp, there were only a handful of camps for children with cancer in existence. The childhood cancer community was only beginning to understand the impact of childhood cancer and its treatment on the child and family. Camps were a new approach to giving children with cancer an opportunity to have a normal childhood experience. There was no data on how to mitigate the impact of a life-threatening diagnosis on a child's development or social and emotional well-being. For me, it felt like the right thing to do—give these kids an opportunity to be with others experiencing the same thing, in a safe setting where they could be "just kids."

Today, research shows the positive impact of summer camp on children with cancer and their families. Since Camp Sunshine began, there are hundreds of pediatric oncology camps nationally and internationally. I encourage you to make a connection with a camp in your area and give local families fighting cancer an opportunity to forge connections and community that might last a lifetime.

Resources

To learn more about Camp Sunshine, visit www.mycampsunshine.com.

Camp Sunshine was a founding member of Children's Oncology Camping Association, International. To learn more about COCA-I or to locate a camp in your area, visit www.cocai.org.

Camp Sunshine was a founding partner of Camp Twin Lakes (CTL), where Camp Sunshine's summer camp and many weekend camp programs are held. To learn more about CTL, visit www.camptwinlakes.org.

To learn more about the Aflac Cancer and Blood Disorders Center at Children's Healthcare of Atlanta, visit www.choa.org/cancer.